The Thin Woman's Brain

Rewiring the Brain for

Permanent Weight Loss

Dilia Suriel

Release 4: February 2014

I.S.B.N. 0-9744092-7-8

Published by:

> Applied Insight, Inc.
> A Colorado Based Corporation

Visit our website:

www.thinwomanbrain.com
Library of Congress cataloging-in publication data:
Suriel, Dilia

The Thin Woman's Brain: Rewiring the Brain for Permanent Weight Loss/4

Topics:

1. Weight Loss
2. Rewiring for Weight Loss
3. Neuroplasticity
4. Cognitive Behavioral Therapy for Weight Loss
5. Alternatives to Dieting
6. Self-Help
7. Lifelong Weight Loss
8. CBT for Weight Loss
9. CBT and Dieting
10. Holistic Weight Loss

It is my belief that humanity will evolve because of female
consciousness.
Too much of our potential is squandered when
so many women feel ashamed of their bodies.
If just 2% of this wasted energy could be rechanneled
toward positive activities,
our entire race would be richly blessed.

Dilia Suriel

Table of Contents

Chapter 1 – Restore the Brain, Lose the Weight

Wired to Overeat

Every year over 10,000 diet books hit the market. Unfortunately 90% of these books are just shuffling the deck chairs on the Titanic. They are:

a) Atkins with a new lipstick,
b) Paleo Paleo Paleo, or
c) So challenging that if you could exert the energy required by the regimen, you would lose weight by the sheer effort necessary to follow the diet.

But here is the most important statistic that anyone considering losing weight should know. Most of the people who manage to lose weight by dieting gain the weight back within the first year! This even includes people who have participated in "The Biggest Loser" or had their stomach stapled. This is the most repressed statistic in the diet industry: only 3 out of every 100 people who reach their goal manage to maintain that weight loss beyond the first year. Take a minute to consider the consequences of that statistic:

Visualize yourself as part of a group of 100 enthusiastic, committed people, who through food restriction and significant exercise manage to burn more calories than they consume each day. Now visualize that this group has the perseverance and stamina to stick to that regimen for months, doing whatever is necessary, AND all of the members of this admirable group actually reach their target weight. Hurray! What an amazing achievement!

One year later these 100 extraordinary people reconvene, and to their shock, only three remain at their weight-loss goals. The other 97 have either returned to the weight they were at prior to the regimen or actually weigh more than when they started the program! Only three – THREE – not even nine, but three, have managed to keep the weight off!

Are we really that spineless? Do we really lack that much willpower? Or is there another explanation? If you conducted a debriefing with the 97 people who could not hang on to their hard-won weight loss, what you would find is that after they attempted to go back to *normal eating,* they experienced hunger far more often than before the weight-loss program. After ending the diet, they also became preoccupied, even obsessed, with food.

There is a little-known organization named the National Weight Control Registry. Their database tracks individuals that have managed to maintain over 30 pounds of weight loss for more than twelve months. The objective of this organization is to learn why certain individuals are able to hold on to their weight loss. In December 2011, *The New York Times* published an article where they interviewed some of these extraordinary individuals. The successful dieters shared how they have to be hypervigilant to maintain their ideal weight. Many of them still have to count calories every single day; some of them even call ahead to restaurants before they attempt a meal out. *The Times* reported that for these individuals, weight maintenance efforts are as much work as losing the weight in the first place. It is a time-consuming, carefully planned, lifelong commitment, predicated on unwavering willpower. Far from peaceful thinness, it is very hard work. Even spokespersons for national weight-loss companies report that the effort required to *keep* the weight off is as significant as the effort exerted to *lose* it.

Now ponder this question: Why is there a need for an entire organization to track those who have managed to maintain their weight loss? At a national level! What does that convey to you about our current methods of losing weight?

Let's examine one simple fact. There was a time in our lives when maintaining a healthy weight was not a struggle. There was a time when we were lean without counting anything. There was a time when we didn't obsess about food. There was a time when we didn't eat compulsively. How are we different from women who don't have these types of food struggles and are thin? That was the pivotal question that changed my life!

Let me introduce myself. I was trained as a scientist and majored in physics and mathematics at a prestigious university. After graduating, I pursued a master's degree, first in electrical engineering and finally settling on computer science. For my entire professional career I worked in the computer industry in jobs ranging from interface engineer to professor of programing languages, culminating at director-level international consulting engagements. I have a track record of solving complex corporate problems and have worked in eight distinct cultures. And while I'm not looking to impress you with my credentials, I do want to share that I'm a world-class analyst. I just happened to wake up one day knowing that I needed to use my analytical talents to end the dieting hell that I'd lived for too many years.

Until the age of 26, I was naturally thin. Then for three years, I invested my hopes, my dreams and fourteen hours a day, seven days a week in my own business. I gained forty pounds during that period of time. Forty pounds! When I finally emerged from the grind of the new business, I put my energy into losing weight. With compulsive weight training and dieting I shed the forty pounds.

But something within me was no longer satisfied with my "normal" weight. Even though I had bludgeoned myself back to my original weight, I was now seduced by my newfound weight-losing skill; I was now shooting for the look of the *latest idol*. My models were no longer the voluptuous bodies of the movie stars of the 1960s, like Raquel Welch, Brigitte Bardot, and Ursula Andress. My new ideal had morphed into … Twiggy, whose body looked like an undernourished teenage boy. I stayed in diet mode because I no longer felt good about my weight. My ideal had transfigured from a size 12 to a size 3, and I couldn't experience myself as attractive in a size 8.

The cycle of gaining weight/losing weight/gaining weight remained for most of my adult life. I believed that the right tools would help me eat less and move more – you know the mantra. I believed what my helpful friends said, that all I needed was BETTER INFORMATION about food and exercise! But in reality I was an expert on all of that. The worst part was the self-hatred: I was "La Gordita," the fat woman. I felt drained. My self-loathing undermined the faith I needed to lose weight. The oppressive shame of living as a fat woman was emotionally damaging. But I never gave up. I continued to diet because, like most of the population, I believed that was my only option – until I noticed that thin women were different, and I flashed back on my pre-diet days.

More Food, Less Pleasure

In the past 10 years, science has made significant progress in understanding why it is so difficult for chronic dieters to achieve long-term weight loss. Our flavor-enhanced food, unrealistic body images, frantic lifestyles, and chronic dieting have caused our brains to change. We've become food-obsessed and depleted our limited willpower to resist the plethora of temptations all around us. We use food to soothe ourselves in the midst of hectic activity, and when we eat, we do so compulsively. These brain-level changes have been documented via imaging technologies. Scientists can now measure statistically significant differences between obese and naturally thin populations. When both groups eat appetizing foods, the amount of dopamine produced in the brain of an obese person is lower than the amount produced in a naturally thin person. Dopamine is experienced as pleasure, so contrary to popular belief, an obese person experiences *less* pleasure from food than her thin counterpart. The obese person needs to eat more food to experience the same amount of pleasure as the thin person.

Despite the popular misconception that obese people love and get greater joy from food, the truth is that the more severe the food addiction, the less pleasure the food addict experiences when eating. This is graphically depicted in the "Brain Reward Center" functional MRI (fMRI) images below, part of a study conducted jointly by Gene-Jack Wang, M.D., Head of Medicine at Brookhaven National Laboratory, and Nora Volkow, M.D., Director of the National Institute on Drug Abuse.

These fMRIs compare the brains of a naturally thin person (on the left) to an obese person (on the right) when eating the same food. The red in the scan of the thin person's brain indicates a high dopamine level, which translates into a healthy dosage of pleasure. In contrast, the red in the obese person's brain indicates a lower dopamine level: the amount of pleasure experienced is substantially less. These images show that the obese person is able to experience less pleasure when eating the same food.

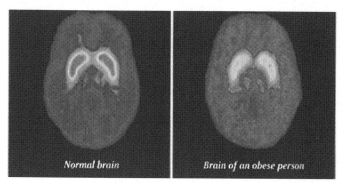

Normal brain   *Brain of an obese person*

Figure 1 - Dopamine Difference, Normal vs. Obese Brains (Red = Dopamine)
Visit thinwomanbrain.com/BookImages for a color version of these fMRIs.

Famine Brain

From the perspective of human evolution, dieting is a last-second phenomenon. It was a mere blip in the 1920s, and it was not until the late 1960s that as a society, as a species, we began repetitive cycles of dieting that triggered the famine-brain mechanism.

Our ancestors adapted to periods of food scarcity by eating as much as possible when food was plentiful. The modern result is that diets prime the brain's reward system for overeating behavior. Weight-loss dieting, by definition, requires reducing food intake below what the body needs to maintain its present form. Although there is no real food scarcity, all of the built-in mechanisms that ensure our survival register a drop in calorie consumption. Researchers are finding, to their dismay, that *any* kind of weight loss deploys our personal neurochemical arsenal and triggers the imperative to eat.

The body, it seems, doesn't "know" when it's storing too much fat; it only "knows" when it's in jeopardy of losing fat. So, in a valiant attempt to regain homeostasis, our system lowers our levels of the hormone that indicate satiety, leptin, and pumps the hunger hormone, ghrelin, into the bloodstream. We call these mechanisms *famine brain* for short. Scientists still don't know exactly how the brain- and physical-hunger systems interact to support or override each other. What we do know is that for many, chronic dieting results in a brain that is food-obsessed.

Restoring the Healthy Brain

While the causes of obesity are numerous, the common thread among them is plasticity of the brain, also called neuroplasticity. As the brain adapts to modern lifestyles – which include stress, overabundance of food, and flavor-enhanced products – it is changed. The good news is that we have also learned to take advantage of neuroplasticity to "rewire" the brain to its healthy state. We *are* able to restore it.

This new form of rehabilitation is called Cognitive Behavioral Therapy (CBT). It is a widely accepted therapy used by psychologists around the world and has been employed successfully to treat obsessive-compulsive disorder, depression, addiction, and various other issues. This book provides step-by-step instructions on how to apply CBT to restore your natural brain, that of a thin woman.

There are four basic steps:

1. Learn to differentiate brain hunger from physical hunger.
2. Observe the brain hunger.
3. Name the real need and address it.
4. Experience success and measure progress.

In contrast to brain hunger, physical hunger has tangible, objective signs: your stomach grumbles, your blood-sugar level is low, you would welcome a variety of foods to end the physical hunger. Brain hunger typically craves very specific foods and its one physical sign, salivation, is usually triggered by external events. Step 1 is the willingness and courage to name the two types of hunger. "I have zero evidence of physical hunger, but I'm craving food. I'm experiencing *brain* hunger."

In Step 2 we observe the symptoms of the addiction. For us, food is like the suave car salesman who is a friend only because he wants us to buy a car. Using several Cognitive Behavioral Therapy techniques, we learn to redirect our entrenched thought patterns. We must recognize the pleasure hallucination for what it is, our current wiring. Incorporating mindfulness practices, we learn to witness our craving and our old belief that food is going to make us feel better. In contrast to willpower, this step is where we calmly observe the craving but are not compelled to act on it.

In Step 3 we name the real need. Are we tired, stressed, disappointed, angry, frustrated, or what? Do we need to take a break, go for a run, express disappointment, in other words, acknowledge an emotional need and address it instead of stuffing it with food?

In Step 4 we continuously recognize our successes, appreciate our progress, and move forward. The human psyche dictates that we must experience progress to continue any long journey. The last step of restoring the brain from that of a food addict to its healthy relationship with food is not only a function of the level of food addiction but also how much pleasure we are able to experience as we progress. The less severe the food addiction and the more pleasure we experience as we recognize our progress, the shorter the rewiring process. Conversely, acute addiction and an inability to experience the pleasure of progress will slow the rewiring process.

There is no diet prescribed in this book, although we do show that foods with flavor-enhancers, high sugar content, or high salt content are addictive. Ending food addiction will mean ending consumption of these types of food. The step-by-step programs in this book will restore your brain to a healthy relationship with food. It is not about overpowering your desire for food. Success is not dependent on willpower. You will learn how you inadvertently allowed food to become way too important in your life and how to regain a healthy perspective toward it.

This book is an invitation to women like me, who for many years followed the yellow brick road, enticed by a magical diet, but were never able to remain in the Emerald City. As with all universal stories, you may recognize yourself in its mirror. If you do, my sincerest wish is that your reflection will also set you free. I'm profoundly moved by this new path; the damaging shame that has weighed my soul down is finally over! Let's embark on this journey together.

Chapter 1 Summary

Our chronic struggle to lose weight is caused by the dieting cycle and other factors that have modified our brains to become food-obsessed. The issue is not to find a novel way to lose weight; most of us are experts on that topic. The real issue is why many of the women who lose weight can eat sensibly only through Herculean, white-knuckle efforts. Based on my personal experience of the weight-loss roller coaster, I know that you have lived through many disappointments, and watched in horror as your hard-won weight goals evaporated in a matter of weeks after many, many months of hard work.

We briefly mentioned the science of neuroplasticity and why it is that we live in craving mode, swinging between starvation and bingeing. The objective of this work is not to change our behavior to mimic a Naturally Thin Woman, nor to adopt her thinking or beliefs, but to return to *feeling* about food the way a Naturally Thin Woman does.

I finally understand how we can comprehensively end the dieting madness. I'm going to share my experience, backed by the latest scientific studies, that returning to our Naturally Thin Woman's brain is the foundation for lifelong and peaceful thinness. The rest of this book is an invitation for you to reclaim your Naturally Thin Woman's brain, and it includes the tools to return to peaceful thinness.

This page has been intentionally left blank.

Chapter 2 – The Thin Woman's Brain

Introduction

My journey toward _The Thin Woman's Brain_ began during the last evening of a get-together with lifelong friends. I took a long walk with a Naturally Thin Woman, my dear friend Alexandra. We had a meaningful history of trust and intimate communication. I shared with Alexandra the deconstruction of my life on the diet maze. I then followed with the disbelief that, once again, I had regained all of the weight I had lost plus additional pounds. At this point Alexandra's eyes teared up. My friend truly loved me, and she was saddened by the fact that not only had I lived through such demoralizing experiences but that they had profoundly damaged my sense of personhood. Being overweight was such a foreign concept for her. She simply did not understand how someone with my tenacity, intelligence, means, and "Navy-Seal willpower" could live the emotional hell that was my life on endless diets.

For all of her adult life, Alexandra had been a size 6. She loved to cook, she ate whatever she wanted, and even though she was a mature woman, she (unlike most American women) had never, ever been on a diet. I was genuinely interested in what made Alexandra _naturally thin_. She was the first of many Naturally Thin Women who agreed to answer all of my questions regarding their relationships with food.

Naturally Thin Versus Will-Powered Thin

I would like to make a critical distinction between Naturally Thin Women like Alexandra and women like my other friend Piper, who through willpower, self-denial, and strict routines, experience long periods of thinness. What I observed is that there is a discernible difference between these two types of women: Alexandra has a healthy relationship with food, in contrast to Piper, who maintains thinness through compulsive calorie-counting, excessive exercising, and a life centered on her preoccupation with staying thin at any cost. I knew Piper's strategies awfully well, as I had achieved many periods of thinness via those same fanatical methods.

The tools used by Will-Powered Thin Women – such as smaller plates, a strict eating regimen, counting every calorie, and drinking massive amounts of water – are all meaningful aids and can be leveraged as helpful stepping stones. This book, however, is not about giving you more diet tricks; you can find plenty of those in most women's magazines. When we don't take the time to address the cause of the dieting rollercoaster, we end up relying on crutches. Crutches are meant to be discarded when the injury is healed. When weight loss is predicated on the use of aids, it is temporary and fleeting.

Furthermore natural thinness is not a function of willpower. As demonstrated by the studies we will discuss later in this book, willpower is limited and is depleted by our many external demands and by our emotional challenges.

What Is a Neural Net?

The central nervous system (which includes the brain and spinal cord) is made up of two basic types of cells: neurons and glia. Neurons are the information messengers. They are the structures by which different areas of the brain communicate. The brain is the central switchboard that transmits messages to the nervous system. Every thought and feeling can be correlated to brain activity.

Figure 2 shows 4 photographs depicting the growth of human neural circuitry. The first photo is the baseline; it shows mostly isolated neurons. The second reflects approximately 60% growth in the number of neurons after 3 months. Photograph 3, taken after 15 months, depicts the beginning of interconnectivity and resembles a young plant root system. In the final photo we see a complex network similar to a metropolitan street map or a mature root system.

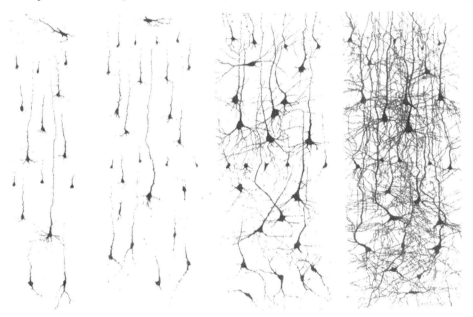

Figure 2 - Growth of Neural Nets

As we learn new skills, our brain's wiring becomes increasingly complex and interconnected.

As someone who for many, many years maintained an overeating lifestyle, I now know that there is a substantial amount of neural circuitry supporting those behaviors. One way to think about these neural nets is that they are part of the organic program that triggers hunger. Imagine that the individual neurons are housed in a brand new suburban development. There are no sidewalks or streets connecting them yet. Then, as neighbors discover each other, they begin to wear paths between their houses. Each time we repeat a behavior, we create more connections between point A and point B in our brain. We are then more likely to take that path again when presented with the same trigger. What we have learned is that we can restore the neural nets that lead to healthier eating behaviors. With practice we strengthen the healthy neural nets and gradually extinguish our old programing.

The Thin Woman's Brain

I want to make the distinction that our focus is not just learning to *think* like a thin woman. We are introducing a process that will cause biological, brain-level changes that can be measured by CAT scans and MRIs. This process will restore the Naturally Thin Woman neural nets that allow us to feel satiated, even in the presence of a sumptuous feast. It is not just about a coping tool like calling a friend or, in our case, running to the refrigerator every time we face a stressful challenge.

Many of us have experienced periods of being able to resist the most enticing smorgasbord while in the initial stages of love. The transformation we are suggesting is not emotional in nature either; it is not trumping one longing with another. This is essentially what goes on in Will-Powered Thin Women's brains, where one force – the desire to overeat – is overpowered by a stronger one – the desire to stay thin. Many of us are able to sustain this suppression mechanism, but only when we have sufficient emotional energy to overpower our voracious appetites.

I've lived the Will-Powered Thin Woman's regimen, and what I know for sure is that the moment the small plate is not available or the lover disappears, or life feels stressful, then I, like most women, resort to overeating. What we'll present in this book is a rewiring of the brain, the restoration of the Naturally Thin Woman's neural nets, where we cultivate the behaviors that lead to a healthy relationship with food. This is not an act of willpower, nor an intellectual construct; we are developing a self-sustaining cycle where modifying behaviors and beliefs changes the organic structures in our brain. This cycle then reinforces the new behaviors and beliefs and brings us to a place where we no longer equate overeating with pleasure.

The goal is to move from the cerebral understanding of concepts to the Sacred YES! This is the intimate moment, when we can acknowledge the pleasure of food *and* have the capacity to accept it *without* an overwhelming compulsion to indulge in it.

At a biological level the Naturally Thin Woman's wiring is different; it is organic, which leads to trust and generates brain signals without stress. In contrast, the Will-Powered Thin Woman's relationship with food is one of internal conflict and negotiations. There is wisdom in Naturally Thin Women's wiring that allows them to simultaneously accept the pleasure of food and peacefully choose to forfeit or postpone that pleasure to the time when they are next hungry.

Let's be crystal clear regarding women who eat like Alexandra versus women who eat like Piper. There are *physiological* differences between Alexandra's brain and Piper's brain – those who are *naturally* thin versus those who *work* relentlessly at being thin. Thin at the price of high stress and willpower is a recipe that we have all tried and that has consistently failed. There are healthy and viable options to lose weight once and for all.

Key Characteristics of Naturally Thin Women

For the past two decades the field of neuroplasticity, the science behind rewiring the brain, has had consistent success in helping people with a range of challenges from alcohol or drug addiction to depression to obsessive-compulsive behavior. These success stories juxtaposed with how Naturally Thin Women relate to food prompted my two crucial questions:

1. What exactly are the brain-level differences between "naturally thin" women and chronic overeaters? And more importantly:
2. Can we rewire our brains to experience food like a Naturally Thin Woman?

With these two questions I embarked upon the final leg of my journey toward peaceful thinness. My first task was to interview several Naturally Thin Women. After multiple interviews of women as diverse as the rainbow – from a street vendor to a former U.S. Congresswoman, from a high school dropout to a college professor, from stay-at-home moms to senior executives – I found nine key characteristics that *most of them* (not all) shared:

1. Most Naturally Thin Women do not obsess about food; only *physical hunger* prompts them to eat.
2. Most Naturally Thin Women enjoy food, but it is not the obsessive love affair experienced by most overeaters.
3. Most Naturally Thin Women make time to enjoy their meals.
4. Most Naturally Thin Women can assess their body needs against their food options.
5. Most Naturally Thin Women dislike the physical discomfort of being bloated or stuffed.
6. Most Naturally Thin Women eat whatever they want while considering the impact of calories.
7. Most Naturally Thin Women do not believe that food is their primary source of joy.
8. Most Naturally Thin Women are attuned with nature.
9. Most Naturally Thin Women have the ability to experience the ups and downs of life.

Let's dig deeper into these nine key characteristics and contrast them to those of chronic dieters.

1. Most Naturally Thin Women do not obsess about food; only *physical hunger* prompts them to eat.

For many years my delusion was that Naturally Thin Women dreamt about carrots and apples while I fantasized about pizza and ice cream. After I became food obsessed, there wouldn't be a period of more than 40 minutes in my typical day when I wasn't contemplating breakfast, planning a morning snack, scheduling lunch, strategizing an afternoon snack, arranging a light dinner, and then rewarding myself with a late evening snack. If I could not sleep, I knew that stuffing myself would help me fall asleep. I was "hungry" most of the time. Food was the pleasure of my life. Food was the dependable friend that would energize me, allow me to power through physical limitations to complete my work, soothe me, and give me an excuse to get together with friends. Food was constantly and permanently on my mind. Food had become my lover.

In contrast, for Naturally Thin Women, food is a physical necessity. At a physiological level their brains are not generating neurotransmitters that fuel the pleasure of anticipation. Their feeling about food is similar to how most of us feel about filling the car with gas. Some of us fill our tanks every Sunday night, others as soon as it gets to the ¼-tank mark, and there are those who wait until the engine is running on fumes. Most overeaters seldom experience true hunger – like hearing our stomachs growl or feeling out of sorts because our blood-sugar level is a bit low. We think about food around the clock, taking every possible excuse to snack and dine and eat again. Our obsession with food grabs us like an emotional undertow and repeatedly drags us away from the shoreline of healthy eating.

Biologically, the overeater's brain is food-obsessed, which is not natural for human beings. Diet restrictions affect the neural nets in the appetite-control center of the brain and lead to what has been termed "famine brain," the driving obsession that locks our brain into compulsive longing for food. So, paradoxically, dieting is the perfect mechanism for generating the food obsession that is characteristic of most overeaters. And how does this obsessive, persistent brain state develop?

One of our fundamental biological imperatives is to nourish ourselves. Whenever the body experiences a drop in blood-sugar level or registers a lower fat content, it triggers a small army of hormones that we experience as overwhelming and compulsive mandates to eat. Within our brains lie receptors wired so that once the brain is in famine mode it drives us to overeat. The biological intent of these mechanisms is to be able to endure periods of food shortages. When our bodies register a drop in body fat or we experience low sugar levels, our brains are wired to deploy a battalion of neurotransmitters, hormones, and chemical mediators that prompt us to avoid famine. These mechanisms evolved over thousands of years to ensure our survival. The glitch is that the brain cannot differentiate between a body with excess fat and a body that has depleted its fat stores and is truly starving. The survival mechanisms that compel us to overeat are triggered by even the smallest drop in body fat.

Food obsession also stems from the suppression mechanism that restricts or forbids certain foods and encourages others. When we diet, we forbid ourselves from having fat, sugar, carbohydrates or whatever it is that we are not supposed to eat during the diet. Harvard School of Medicine's Daniel Wegner, Ph.D., conclusively demonstrated that telling our brain *not* to think about a specific item is the most effective way to make the brain obsess about it. This mechanism has been demonstrated in the challenge, "For the next 60 seconds do not think about a polar bear." This restriction – and it can be carbs, fat, sugar, calories or whatever food category we are avoiding this year – is the phenomenon that Wegner termed the "ironic monitoring process," popularly known as the *Polar Bear Effect.*

Most of us have experienced that diets work only under ideal conditions; in other words, when we are hypervigilant, rested, and relaxed. It is only then that our suppression mechanism can override the obsession that makes us want to eat. However, as soon as we are stressed or challenged, whenever our willpower is depleted, we immediately seek out the very substance that we have been suppressing. Anyone who has ever been on a diet knows that willpower is not an unlimited resource.

A key study jointly conducted at the University of Florida, the University of Utah, and Case Western Reserve demonstrated that most human beings have a limited supply of self-control, and after continual demand, that supply can dry up. The scientists termed this phenomenon *ego depletion*. In Freudian psychology the ego is the part of our personality that mediates between what we want and what we think is appropriate. The ego keeps you from eating the entire cheesecake at a party because you don't want others to think you are a glutton. The researchers determined that any task requiring self-control can have a hindering effect on a subsequent task also requiring self-control, even if these tasks are completely unrelated.

The "ego depletion" studies have been critical in disproving the commonly held notion that there is infinite willpower and that the issue with most women who don't adhere to their diets is *lack* of willpower.

2. Most Naturally Thin Women enjoy food, but it is not the obsessive love affair experienced by most overeaters.

Once a Naturally Thin Woman experiences physical hunger, she selects what she will eat; choosing food is not an obsessive or fantastic reverie. Whenever I used to think about food, my brain lit up like a pin-ball machine. Whereas a Naturally Thin Woman derives sensory pleasure *in her body* from the physical act of eating, my greatest pleasure was *in my head.* I fantasized about food; I daydreamed about whatever amazingly delicious treats I was going to eat – sometime soon. This has recently been substantiated by scientists studying the reward hotspots in the brain: the anticipation of the food generates dopamine, the neurotransmitter associated with pleasure. The food-obsessed brain is functioning differently.

Think of it this way. Suppose you've met someone that you feel overpoweringly attracted to, so much that you spend days or weeks fantasizing about the idyllic romantic encounter that will transpire the next time your paths cross. And then you actually spend time with this man and your impeccably scripted plan becomes a terribly awkward exchange. It leaves you feeling disillusioned and wondering how on earth you convinced yourself that this man was your perfect mate. The food-obsessed brain invests a great deal of time planning the next eating rendezvous and, in most cases, the act of consuming the food is not as satisfying as the fantasy.

Naturally Thin Women do not tell themselves that in order to continue being thin they cannot eat specific foods. This is perhaps one of the most surprising differences between the wiring of a Naturally Thin Woman like Alexandra and a Will-Powered Thin Woman like Piper. Alexandra thoroughly enjoys bread, butter, and fat-laden foods, trusting that she will stop indulging in them when her body tells her that it is satiated. Piper will avoid these foods like the plague because the *diet du jour* says she is not supposed to eat them.

For the Naturally Thin Woman, there is no struggle or emotional charge around eating, or for that matter around having fattening food in the house. There is no love-hate relationship with food, no negotiating with it. Eating is a pleasure, a sensual joy; it is wonderfully satisfying.

Because of the Polar Bear Effect most overeaters have a short sprint of sublime adherence to a specific set of eating regimens, followed by an explosive burst of bingeing or long periods of "I don't give a shit" – stuffing themselves with whatever food bears the label "I'm-not-supposed-to-eat-this." Their relationship with food runs the gamut from iron-willed self-control to a frenzied, all-bets-are-off tornado.

3. Most Naturally Thin Women make time to enjoy their meals.

There is nothing more delicious than eating a meal when we have a genuine appetite. Our taste buds are alive; we are able to experience flavors, discern textures, and fully delight in aromas. Physical hunger has specific body signals and sensations – our mouths water at the sight of food; we have heightened sensations of texture in our cheeks, teeth, tongue, and upper palate; our stomach rumbles; we experience low blood-sugar levels. From these awakened body sensations, most Naturally Thin Women experience *physical hunger*, and it is then that they begin to plan what would feel good to eat.

I spoke with several Naturally Thin Women who shared how they experience the act of eating. They talk about preparing a beautiful meal; they use words like *symphony, velvety, luscious, silky, kaleidoscope, stimulating, explosion.* Eating is an enchanting love affair – unhurried, present, and explorative, even seductive. In fact, they would rather *not* eat than hurry through the experience, perhaps just grabbing a small snack to tide them over. In contrast it used to take me three minutes flat from the time the food was in front of me to the time it was gone. I ate like a piranha. Unlike Alexandra, there was no courting, no preparation, no planning, no first date; it was locate, acquire, devour.

Once food becomes an obsession, we attempt to fulfill the mental spectacle that has been marinating for hours prior to the physical act of eating. So by the time the food was in front of me, the actual experience of eating could never match the fantasy that had been indulged in my mind. The brain chemistry that was generating pleasure during my food fantasy was more pleasurable than the physical eating experience.

The wiring to fully experience food explains why many Naturally Thin Women "forget to eat" when their lives are in chaos; they don't experience pleasure in hurrying through a meal, as it is inconsistent with fully enjoying it. Setting time aside to enjoy a meal is a stark contrast to the three-minute "fast foods" or "eating on the run" that many of the rest of us call eating. Once we understand famine brain, we understand why, for most overeaters, hunger feels like an overwhelming imperative that fuels a compulsion never experienced by Naturally Thin Women.

4. Most Naturally Thin Women can assess their body needs against their food options.

A Naturally Thin Woman trusts the messages from her body and honors its desires; if she wants a piece of cheesecake or pizza, she will eat it. In contrast, many of us have stopped trusting our body messages and have been convinced that only by completely forfeiting entire categories of foods will we have a chance of losing weight.

A Naturally Thin Woman will not eat food that does not appeal to her. What's the point? If she doesn't like her choices, her internal dialogue goes like this: "If my only options are yucky food, I'd rather have a snack until I can sit down and enjoy what I truly want." Or if she really doesn't have the time to eat she will say to herself, "I'd rather postpone my meal; I don't enjoy rushing through the experience." Yes, genuine hunger will drive her to eat, but only if it's a positive experience; she is not driven by *famine brain,* and her choices are not propelled by overpowering compulsion. Once she becomes physically hungry, Alexandra is very specific as to what she prefers to eat. With a healthy mind-body connection, unimpeded by the fear of being FAT, Alexandra has access to her hunger needs and can clearly express them:

- I am hungry.
- This doesn't appeal to me.
- That looks really yummy!
- Yuck, that doesn't taste good – I'm not eating any more of it.
- I am thirsty, not hungry.

Trusting her body messages is in huge contrast to thin women like Piper who are constantly negotiating calories, which then fuels an internal argument with her innate desires:

- That's all I'm supposed to eat, and damn it, I'm not eating any more.
- I will NOT allow myself to be FAT.
- It's only two more hours before I can eat – I will force myself to wait it out.
- I'll drink water until it's time to eat.
- I'll do something else to distract myself.

These are important distinctions; the Naturally Thin Woman trusts her appetite, what sounds good to eat, and her desire to enjoy the meal. She also knows that having to rush through a meal is not pleasurable, and so she would rather eat a snack and wait until she has the time to enjoy the meal. She eats with the confidence and trust that she will not gain weight.

5. **Most Naturally Thin Women dislike the physical discomfort of being bloated or stuffed.**

In fact, the word consistently used by Naturally Thin Women to describe the feeling of being stuffed was HATE. "I HATE feeling stuffed." "I don't care if I'm eating with the Queen of England at the most sumptuous gourmet feast on the planet. Once I am full, nothing will make me overeat." Someone once attempted to entice Alexandra to finish what was left on her plate, and she responded, "I don't give a shit if there is food on the plate. I'm not a garbage can; I'm FULL."

Alexandra once told me that she thinks of her stomach as being the size of a softball and she knows that filling it beyond its limits has negative consequences:

- I feel like I'm tied down – a lead balloon, uncomfortable in my clothes.
- I feel hostage to my body; it limits my ability to do so many other activities.
- My range of movement is limited, and simple activities, like walking up stairs, are miserable.
- It compromises the quality of my life.
- If I really like the taste of something and I'm full, I can have more later … when I'm not full and I can enjoy it. Duh.

Being full was a foreign concept to me. I always ate whatever was on the plate, I always went for seconds, and I always, *always* wanted dessert … often my reward for going without bread, or for eating greens. The idea of being full occurred only when I had stuffed myself so grossly that it was physically unbearable to move. I would not stop until I felt disgust and shame and physically could not eat any more.

Another notable difference between Naturally Thin Women and Will-Powered Thin Women is the ability to trust their body messages, to recognize once they are satiated. I once asked Alexandra how she can tell when she's full. The answer was so simple it floored me. "The food loses its taste. It doesn't taste as good as when I began eating. The taste becomes bland." Women like Alexandra can discern when they are full; they trust the signals that their bodies generate. That complete trust, that absence of anxiety, allows us to eat without compulsion.

Once I began eating like a Naturally Thin Woman, I no longer worried about being sleepy in the afternoon because I ate too much at lunch. I am now able to enjoy much more of life because I am not recuperating from a large meal. I can go dancing or on a brisk walk right after dinner because I'm not down for the evening. Knowing and trusting the sensation of fullness has increased the quality of my life significantly.

6. Most Naturally Thin Women eat whatever they want while considering the impact of calories.

Eating the way Naturally Thin Women eat, if I have a desire for a sub, pizza, fettuccini Alfredo, Haagen-Dazs® or chocolate, I will honor that desire and have that exact food. I don't worry about overeating because I have learned how to eat mindfully (more on this in Chapter 4), and I know that the taste of the food will not be as enticing once my body has had enough. I savor every bite, but I stop eating the moment it loses its taste. Eating the *entire carton* of ice cream no longer has any appeal.

Alexandra shared with me her internal dialogue, which goes something like this; "Yes, I could have this donut because it is sitting right here in front of me, but I'd rather eat that luscious piece of chocolate that I really, truly want." Forfeiting the donut because we prefer to eat chocolate is an example of the distinction between choice and self-deprivation.

Naturally Thin	Will-Powered Thin
"I choose"	"I will make myself"
"I prefer"	"I can't have"
"I'd rather"	"It's not in my diet"

In a University of Houston study, psychologists Vanessa M. Patrick, Ph.D., and Henrik Hagtvedt, Ph.D., demonstrated that there is a higher level of empowerment when we believe we have options. Naturally Thin Women use statements such as "I prefer" to indicate that they are choosing. In contrast, Will-Powered Thin Women act out of a limited set of options so they typically use the expression "I can't." For a Naturally Thin Woman, each calorie has to be worth it, and the brain reacts very differently to a choice than to a denial of our basic desire. Think about people who have an attack dog but they have trained it to be aggressive only when they are in need of protection. Contrast that to people who own dogs that are vicious by nature and have not trained them. These dogs have to be kept muzzled at all times, as they will attack as soon as the muzzle is off. When we constantly control and constrain our eating by sheer willpower, we are like that muzzled dog. Our brains are running the famine-avoidance programing, a biological imperative that drives our compulsion to overeat. It explains why we feel totally out of control during bingeing episodes.

Trusting that we will stop eating when we are full allows us to choose the foods that we find appetizing. Instead of relying on willpower, we need to restore our healthy neural nets; we need to allow the famine-brain wiring to atrophy.

7. Most Naturally Thin Women do not believe that food is their primary source of joy.

I personally know that when I sing, when I dance, when I'm laughing, I forget about food. When I'm doing work that is creative, I'm not hungry. Joy for me is hugging and connecting to another human being at an intimate level. It is letting the music move me and releasing my body into a flow of freedom; it is sharing a common vision, being in a state of grace.

Studies show an irrefutable negative correlation between experiencing joy and the predisposition to addictive behaviors. For example, a Simon Fraser University study, led by psychologist Bruce K. Alexander, Ph.D., documented that when mice lived in their version of nirvana, they were 91% less likely to indulge in drug-laced sugar water. This study, known as "Rat Park," provided an enriched environment for the rats, both physically and socially, with an abundance of balls and wheels for play and enough space for mating and raising litters. Other studies like Rat Park have conclusively demonstrated that the more joyful a person feels, the less likely that person is to support an addiction.

What is important is your own personal experience. When you are engaged in activities that you find joyous, you are less likely to overeat. Part of this work will show you how to identify activities that align you with joy while recognizing those that make you inexplicably hungry. Learning this distinction leads to a life where, instead of searching for food when you are out of balance, you begin to search for true nourishment.

8. Most Naturally Thin Women are attuned with nature.

Artificial lighting became widely available in just the last 100 years of our human history. Before artificial lighting became the standard, the rhythm of our day was dictated by sunrise and sunset. We were part of the natural world and the forces that act upon it, such as the sun and moon.

The Chinese articulated their version of these natural rhythms thousands of years ago. They talked about the rhythmic circulation of Qi (energy), how there was an organized flow of this energy throughout the day from one organ system to the next, how the ebb and flow of this Qi corresponded with different human cycles. For instance, because the stomach and spleen are at their peak function between 7 and 11 A.M., this would be the time for optimal digestion of nutrients. Ayurveda, an ancient Indian system, says that optimum digestion is between 10 A.M. and 2 P.M.

This knowledge correlates with what we today call circadian rhythms, and it is why eating a larger breakfast and lunch and a smaller dinner (when digestive function is slowing down) is optimal for restoring alignment with nature. Interestingly, according to the Chinese, the peak function of the large intestine is 5 to 7 A.M., just prior to the peak time for digestion. This suggests that the natural rhythm is to empty our digestive system in preparation for beginning the cycle all over again.

We have adapted to our societal structures, and many of us have moved our heaviest meal to nighttime. Most Naturally Thin Women whom I interviewed expressed a preference toward eating a light supper and reserving breakfast or lunch for their larger meal.

9. **Most Naturally Thin Women have the ability to experience the ups and downs of life.**

- For a Naturally Thin Woman, disappointment leads to expression; she is able to articulate "I'm disappointed" as opposed to suppressing it with food.
- For a Naturally Thin Woman, sadness leads to tears; she weeps, in contrast to an emotional overeater who raids the refrigerator and then wonders why.
- For a Naturally Thin Woman, anger might lead to throwing plates against the wall, but in most cases she is able to give her anger verbal expression, instead of stuffing her face.
- For a Naturally Thin Woman, being tired means sleep, even if it means a catnap on the floor, or going home for a few hours to rest.
- For a Naturally Thin Woman, loneliness leads to reaching out, talking to a close friend and expressing her loneliness, as opposed to having a date with Mr. Häagen-Dazs®.
- For a Naturally Thin Woman, stress means a long run, a few yoga postures, meditation, or acknowledging what was causing the stress.

Naturally Thin Women have not adopted the pervasive belief that food is a meaningful to feeling good, it is not the primary form of addressing emotional needs. They don't believe that food is a source of comfort, that food will entertain them when they are feeling bored. Food is not a meaningful way to deal with anger. Bottom line, the Naturally Thin Woman's belief system has not endowed food with the emotional healing powers that most overeaters have given it.

Whereas persistent and recurrent emotional imbalances would send most overeaters toward food, Naturally Thin Women face and experience all of the emotions that are part of being human. Once accepted, these emotions need to be felt, expressed, embodied, and finally released – by crying, reaching out to a friend, jogging, or whatever strategy helps us be with our feelings. Eating will only replace the avoidance of the emotion with self-loathing.

In order to end the cycle of "on-a-diet" and recognize it as "on-denial," it is essential to accept and experience our emotions fully.

Chapter 2 Summary

In this chapter we've established the differences between how the Naturally Thin Woman and the Will-Powered Thin Woman experience food. We summarized the nine key characteristics of most Naturally Thin Women and their relationship to food. I hope that you remember the natural and healthy relationship you had with food before your brain became food-obsessed, the healthy and trusting experience that will trump a million diets and tricks. A healthy relationship with food does not mean that the Naturally Thin Woman longs for or eats healthy greens all the time. It means that she has a positive, not antagonistic, relationship to what she eats. To return to our Naturally Thin Woman behaviors requires us to short-circuit our existing wiring.

Some of the practices might be more challenging than others, but like anything that needs to be unlearned, the limiting factor is being willing to step forward after each failure. And then the hypervigilance, the dread of living on perpetual guard against the next snack attack, will be eradicated.

While the brain is incredibly complex, the concept of neural nets is not. Neurons are elongated, branched cells in the brain and other parts of the nervous system. Because of their many branches, multiple neurons can form complex physical networks called neural nets. Information travels along neurons as electrical impulses and is transmitted from one neuron to the next by chemical neurotransmitters. These neural nets are sometimes compared to electrical wiring. Everything we think and feel is the result of transmissions along neural nets.

Neural nets can grow and change over time. The more often a pathway in the network is used, the stronger it becomes. As we learn, new branches and connections form. It's not about willpower. It's about restoring the brain of a Naturally Thin Woman. Read on to learn how.

Chapter 3 – The Food Addict's Brain

Introduction

It was important for me to understand the science behind how my brain became wired to overeat. Understanding helped me stop feeling ashamed for being overweight. It helped me realize what I was up against in trying to eradicate this behavior for the rest of my life. It instilled in me a desire to return to a Naturally Thin Woman instead of continuing to pursue diets that kept me food-obsessed or, at best, a Will-Powered Thin Woman. In this section we summarize the scientific findings on how the brain has been wired for overeating.

The Brain's Pleasure Center

Our pleasure center resides in the center of the brain and is what produces feelings of motivation and reward. Its primary job is to make us feel good or "reward" us when we engage in any behavior that is necessary for survival, such as escaping danger, eating, being nurtured, and procreating. This is a self-reinforcing mechanism because, by repeating these pleasurable behaviors over and over, we not only ensure the survival of the species, we also ensure a sense of well-being and self-worth. Our biology is so magnificent that whenever we execute any of the survival imperatives, the brain produces specialized chemicals that stimulate the pleasure center. Whenever we eat, have sex, or outrun that saber-toothed tiger, we experience a chemical high that we recognize as pleasure and that can be measured in the body as an increased level of the neurotransmitter called *dopamine*. A neurotransmitter is any chemical released by nerve cells to send signals to other nerve cells.

Dopamine was first identified in 1964 by Swedish researchers Annica Dahlström, M.D., and Kjell Fuxe, M.D. But it was not until 1990 that Kenneth Blum, Ph.D., a neuropsychopharmacologist and geneticist, explained that dopamine is dependent on the healthy production of upstream neurotransmitters. The process begins with the generation of the neurotransmitter serotonin, followed by enkephalin, which binds to endogenous opioid receptors. This inhibits the production of GABA, the neurotransmitter that limits dopamine production. In turn, the reduced amount of GABA results in overproduction of dopamine, which in some individuals leads to an unhealthy amount of anxiety.

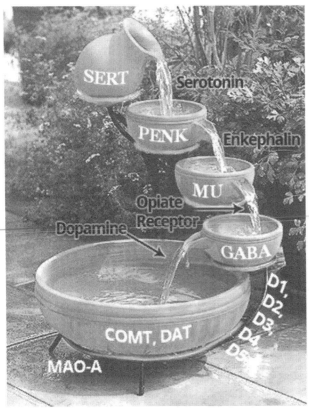
Figure 3 - Healthy Dopamine Production

The amount of each neurotransmitter is determined by the health of its supporting genes. The illustration shows that the generation of serotonin is dependent on the health of the SERT gene, depicted as the pot from which serotonin cascades. The same goes for enkephalin, as it relies on the health of the PENK gene. The endogenous opioid receptors are predicated on the MU gene, and for GABA it is the GabaRAP gene. Even when all of the upstream neurotransmitters are being produced at healthy levels, the genes associated with the production of dopamine receptors, specifically the D1 to D5 and the COMT, DAT and MAO-A genes also need to be healthy.

It's important to understand the complexity of the dopamine mechanism. Any deficiencies or damage to the required genes can affect our ability to experience the "normal" amount of pleasure that we are supposed to feel when we eat.

Famine Brain

The primal imperative for any species is to survive. From an evolutionary perspective, humans lived as hunter-gatherers for hundreds of thousands of years; food supplies were scarce and unpredictable. As hunter-gatherers we had little means of storing food, and no concentrated food sources beyond what we could obtain each day. Our ability to store grains for later consumption did not start until 10,000 years ago when we evolved into farming communities. Beyond salting certain foods our ability to store highly perishable food was not widely available until the 1850s. Under these conditions overeating ensured our survival. In fact, evolution has furnished us with a suite of neurotransmitters and a battalion of hormones to guarantee that we over-consume food in preparation for famine conditions. These neurochemicals and neural circuits make eating a deeply pleasurable activity. We want to eat, frequently even in the absence of metabolic need. The brain-hunger system motivates and rewards eating by creating conscious sensations and impulses related to food: I like that. I want that. That was good. I want more. If your mouth waters when you pass the pastry shop after lunch, you can blame brain hunger. If you find yourself exchanging good cash for a nutritionally deficient profiterole, blame brain hunger.

"Under famine conditions, the ability to ingest and store as many calories as possible when food is readily available would have obvious survival value," observes neurologist Barry E. Levin, M.D., of the New Jersey Medical School in Newark. "The ability to overeat during periods of sporadic feast represented a survival advantage in ancestral societies subjected to periods of starvation. Under scarce and unpredictable conditions, the built-in reward for overeating worked beautifully." Dr. Levin documented in the *Journal of Physiology* that our "biology is metabolically suited to the intermittent availability of food."

Yet if the potency of appetite seems excessive, consider this: How many meals would you skip if you never had any cravings? The answer is probably too many. If eating were an experience as neutral as breathing, would we bother to spend hours each day shopping, cooking, and blowing our paychecks in restaurants? Or would we have to remind ourselves, every so often, to take time out for a bite – the way we sometimes catch ourselves holding our breath and remind ourselves to breathe?

The Food Addict's Brain is Different

How is the food addict's brain different from the Naturally Thin Woman's brain? In this section we will highlight the differences, specifically:

- We are food obsessed.
- We mostly eat in a compulsive manner.
- It takes a lot more food for us to feel satiated.
- We experience "brain" hunger frequently.
- We have stronger responses to food cues.
- Emotional imbalances cause brain hunger.

A functional magnetic resonance imaging machine (fMRI) uses the magnetic properties of blood to measure which brain regions are most active when the subject experiences specific events. Neuroscientists are able to measure brain activities of food addicts when exposed to food cues, when eating tasty foods, or after eating specific foods. "It is similar to working out," Ashley Gearhardt, Ph.D., explains. "When you are working a certain muscle, blood rushes to that area. The brain appears to work the same way, and we can track what brain regions are receiving the most blood."

fMRIs consistently show that the prefrontal cortex is a convergence zone for reward stimuli, particularly experiencing pleasure during eating. To clarify the neurobiological mechanisms that influence appetite, Dr. Gearhardt presented normal-weight and obese subjects with color photographs of foods while they were undergoing an fMRI. These photographs varied from high-reward to low-reward foods. She demonstrated that food-addicted subjects responded to high-reward foods similarly to how addicts respond to drugs.

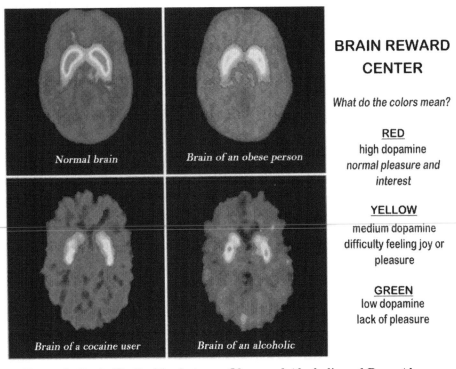

BRAIN REWARD CENTER

What do the colors mean?

RED
high dopamine
normal pleasure and
interest

YELLOW
medium dopamine
difficulty feeling joy or
pleasure

GREEN
low dopamine
lack of pleasure

Normal brain

Brain of an obese person

Brain of a cocaine user

Brain of an alcoholic

Figure 4 - Brain Similarities between Obese and Alcoholic and Drug Abusers
Visit thinwomanbrain.com/BookImages for a color version of these fMRIs.

This illustration contrasts a normal brain with brains of different types of addicts. As you can see, the pleasure center of the obese person shows more similarity to the cocaine user and alcoholic than to the normal brain.

Bart Hoebel, Ph.D., of Princeton University was one of the first to study rats addicted to sugar. He showed that every drop of sugar syrup they swallowed caused a surge in their dopamine levels. Like human addicts, Hoebel's sugar-junkie rats developed hypersensitivity in the dopamine receptors that overreacted to a variety of drugs. The changes were long-term: even after a month of abstinence, the taste of sugar incited the rats to addictive behavior.

In a similar study at the University of Alabama at Birmingham, Mary Boggiano, Ph.D., documented that junk food binges in rats set off the same pleasure receptors in the brain that are stimulated when drug addicts take opiates. Dr. Boggiano's Oreo®-bingeing rats had long-term changes in their brains' endogenous opioids that somehow made them unusually responsive to flavor-enhanced foods.

And, if that cream puff tastes as good as sex feels, that's no coincidence. The dopamine reward system is how we feel pleasure, and it is implicated in compulsive gambling and drug abuse, as well as sex addiction. Eating satisfaction emanates from some of the same neural signals and pathways that orchestrate orgasm. Consequently, hundreds of neuroscientists have begun to document that obesity, eating disorders, and even the ordinary urges of appetite resemble addiction. "Boosting dopamine time after time is what drugs of abuse do," Dr. Hoebel says. "That makes you wonder whether food might have addictive properties." Duh!

"Food gives you a modest physiological response via the same pathways that drugs give you a tremendous response," says psychiatrist Walter H. Kaye, M.D., Director of the eating-disorders program at the University of California in San Diego. "Drugs hijack the food-reward pathways." Drugs have addictive effects because they tap into the appetite's pleasure pathways.

A food fix, like any drug fix, is an attempt to experience the dopamine high craved by any addict. In the 1954 study credited with the identification of the pleasure center, two researchers at McGill University, James Olds, Ph.D., and Peter Milner, Ph.D., documented the effects of dopamine. In this study, rats could push a bar to have the pleasure center electrically stimulated or they could push a bar for food. Drs. Olds and Milner documented that for the rats, electrical stimulation of the pleasure center was more rewarding than food. In fact, the experience was so rewarding that a starving rat would ignore food in favor of the high that was produced by electrically stimulating her pleasure center. Some rats stimulated their brains more than 2,000 times per hour for 24 consecutive hours! In fact, most of the rats died of starvation.

Heroin and cocaine addicts also tend to forget to eat and, while taking their drugs, often lose a lot of weight. This explains why, when we are getting our dopamine fix from other sources – first stages of love, any activity that we find very enjoyable (for me dancing, singing, soulful conversation) – we are less likely to overeat. In fact, we forget to eat! The addiction is not to the food, it's to the dopamine high. When that mechanism is faulty, we become food-obsessed and overeat in an attempt to get our dopamine fix.

Food Obsession

As with most addicts, my drug of choice had an overwhelming power. I remember attending a sumptuous party where, typically, I would overindulge. I brought home a rather enticing piece of chocolate cake, but I was stuffed, so I firmly told myself that I would eat it later. After hours of tossing and turning, the clock read 3:11 A.M. when I finally acquiesced, realizing that I would either have to get up and eat it or not get any sleep resisting the urge.

It was excruciating sharing food family style. Everyone would finish, and the waiter always took too long to pick up the leftovers. I would be mesmerized by the remaining food, to the point of becoming oblivious to the conversations around me.

I could never have my forbidden foods in the house, as they would get eaten within a few hours. If I was at a party where everyone was sitting around the food, I simply could not tolerate being in such close proximity to so many temptations. As food addicts, we obsess about food; when we aren't eating we think about food incessantly.

Dr. Gearhardt, while a fellow at the Rudd Center for Food Policy and Obesity at Yale University, conducted neurobiological studies where she documented the similarities in the way the brain responds to drugs and flavor-enhanced foods. Like drug addicts, people with food addiction struggle with increased cravings and stronger urges when exposed to food cues and may feel more out-of-control when eating something delicious. Even a single morsel of a cookie can trigger a binge, much as a single drink can send an alcoholic on a bender. "The findings of this study support the theory that compulsive eating may be driven in part by an enhanced anticipation of food rewards,"

Dr. Gearhardt stated. Participants with higher food addiction scores showed greater brain activity in areas correlated with cravings, but less activity in the regions responsible for inhibiting urges.

In brain-imaging studies of human subjects, Gene-Jack Wang, M.D., head of medicine at Brookhaven National Laboratory in Upton, New York, and Nora Volkow, M.D., Director of the National Institute on Drug Abuse, have shown that the mere sight and smell of barbecued chicken, hamburgers, and pizza release dopamine in the brain. This food stimulation significantly increases dopamine levels in binge eaters but not in normal eaters. The amount of dopamine released correlates with the strength of the subjects' yearning to eat: the subjective impression of *I want that*. "This is how our brains control our desire," says Dr. Wang. Many food addicts feel powerless about their ability to control when and how much they eat. "Now we're not just talking about energy balance," says Dr. Wang, "We're talking about human psychology."

Compulsive Eating

When I gave away my large clothes I noticed something very significant: not one of them was stain-free! Every single blouse or dress top was splattered with an oil stain or a sauce stain or some other type of food – every single one of them! Eating was a frenzy. I ate with the voracity of a piranha; eating was attempting to get a fix as quickly as humanly possible.

I remember being invited to an exquisitely elegant and expensive all-you-can-eat Easter buffet. I ate two servings for each one that the rest of the party ate. My host noted, "Wow, you are efficient in getting your money's worth." In looking back I'm sure they were alarmed at the gluttony and ferocity of my eating and the very massive amount of food that I was able to consume.

My story is not unique. Most overeaters exhibit a level of anxiety that doesn't allow us to eat in a calm or mindful manner. Because our brains are, biologically speaking, off the tracks and out of control, when we do eat, it is with an intensity that can only be described as compulsive.

In humans, the striatum is activated not only by stimuli associated with reward, but also by aversive, novel, unexpected, or intense stimuli, and cues associated with such events. If you think of the brain as a motor vehicle, then the ventral striatum is the accelerator. When food enters a person's body it stimulates the pleasure center, and the pleasure center in turn increases the flow of dopamine.

When overeating becomes a standard behavior, three things happen: 1) the reward system is hijacked, 2) neuroplastic changes occur, and 3) the neurotransmitter GABA, the "braking system," is decreased. When brakes fail, the train will run away and eventually jump off the tracks. Similarly, food addiction derails the pleasure center; it's all accelerator and no brakes.

Drug Tolerance and Why We Overeat

Eating is one of our biological imperatives, and it has been insured by the pleasure we feel when we eat. However, once we become addicted to food, just as a long-term alcoholic can drink everyone under the table and a drug addict needs larger and larger amounts of drugs, we develop a higher tolerance for food. In all forms of addiction, it takes a continually larger amount of the addictive substance to experience a dopamine high. Chronic drinkers show fewer signs of intoxication even at high blood-alcohol concentrations, which in non-drinkers would be incapacitating or even fatal. Tolerance facilitates the consumption of increasing amounts of alcohol and results in physical dependence. Likewise, the food addict's brain requires more food to generate the amount of dopamine associated with a normal pleasure fix.

One of the most poignant examples of tolerance is men who are addicted to Internet pornography. Once a man is fully addicted to this form of dopamine fix, he reports that he cannot feel excited or satisfied during intercourse with a real woman. It takes him months of abstaining from X-rated sites and withstanding intense withdrawal symptoms before he can regain the experience of pleasure when interacting with an actual woman.

In 2001, Dr. Wang and his colleagues, Dr. Volkow among them, compared the brain scans of obese and normal-weight volunteers, counting up dopamine receptors. Obese people, Dr. Wang realized, had fewer dopamine receptors — the more obese they were, the fewer of these crucial receptors they had. In fact, he said, the brains of obese people and drug addicts look strikingly similar: "Both have fewer dopamine receptors than normal subjects." Every addict is seeking a fix, but when we develop a tolerance for our drug, in our case food, eating smaller amounts of less tasty food leaves us with diminished feelings of pleasure, because the dopamine mechanism has gone amuck.

When a gene that is vital to the dopamine process is damaged, the addict experiences less pleasure from the same amount of the substance that had previously given her a high. Simply stated, we are generating less dopamine, so we overeat in an attempt to achieve our previous level of pleasure. What drives us to overeat is our need for a dopamine fix.

As we discussed in Chapter 1, the notion that an obese woman experiences more pleasure when eating than her thin counterpart is flawed. Once again the fMRI in Figure 5 shows that a healthy brain generates substantially higher amounts of dopamine than the brain of a food addict. Food addiction has the same negative consequences as other addictions; the addict continually builds a higher tolerance for her drug. The lower amount of dopamine implies less pleasure, which then leads most food addicts to consume a significantly higher amount of food – one of the tangible and measurable differences between the brain of a Naturally Thin Woman and her obese counterpart.

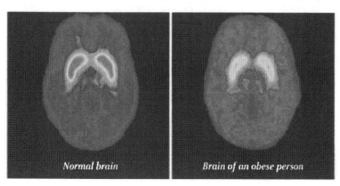

Figure 5 - Dopamine Contrast, Healthy vs. Obese Brains
Visit thinwomanbrain.com/BookImages for a color version of these fMRIs.

This explains why we compulsively eat whenever we fail to reach the anticipated pleasure. We are simply not generating enough dopamine.

Intense Response to Food Cues

Food addicts experience overwhelming hunger in the presence of food cues. Compulsive overeaters are more susceptible to strong cravings after smelling or seeing food, even after a full meal when they are not hungry. Researchers call this phenomenon "external food sensitivity." In a study conducted by scientists at the British Medical Research Council, brain scans revealed how this food sensitivity influences people's eating habits.

The researchers, Andrew Calder, Ph.D., Luca Passamonti, Ph.D., and James Rowe, Ph.D., were trying to determine why some people are more likely to overeat. Published in the *Journal of Neuroscience* (January 2011), the study used brain scans to show how the participants reacted to three sets of images: appetizing food, bland food, and unrelated images of other subjects. "People who appear to be more sensitive to food signals have different wiring in their brains," said obesity expert Marc-Andre Cornier, M.D., a University of Colorado endocrinologist who was not associated with the study.

According to Yale's Dr. Gearhardt, "Addicted individuals are more likely to be physiologically, psychologically, and behaviorally reactive to triggers such as advertising. The possibility that food-related cues may trigger pathological reactions is of special concern in the current food environment, where highly palatable foods are constantly available and heavily marketed." Like drug addicts, people with food addiction may struggle with increased cravings and stronger urges to eat in response to food cues and may feel more out-of-control when eating something delicious. We feel powerless around food, and the sense of "I can't help myself" dominates. This stands in stark contrast to the Naturally Thin Woman who is unaware that this type of struggle is even possible.

Emotional Imbalance Causes Hunger

As a positive person, my strongest allergy was to anything that compromised my optimistic outlook. Anytime my energy level was low, I ate. Stress was mitigated with food; ditto for uncomfortable feelings, challenging situations, difficult people. Anything that took me out of my sunny comfort zone resulted in a trip to the kitchen.

When we are addicted to food, our brains are programmed to use food to temporarily eliminate anxiety, irritability, stress, depression – any uncomfortable feelings – with a dopamine fix. The longer we use food to "feel better," the more likely it is that we associate relief from feeling bad with our addictive substance. When we have a low tolerance for the ups and downs of life, our primary coping mechanism is a dopamine fix; any emotional imbalance equals an overeating episode.

Measurable Brain Differences

Since 2009 studies have irrefutably documented a statistically significant difference between the brains of obese people and those of lean individuals. Below are a few examples of these studies.

A June 2013 fMRI study at the Oregon Research Institute led by Sonja Spoor, Ph.D., and Eric Stice, Ph.D., measured brain differences between obese and lean individuals. The dorsal striatum plays a role in reward, and obese individuals have less active striatal dopamine receptors compared to lean individuals – yet another study that indicates that obese subjects receive less pleasure from the same amount of food.

According to the DANA Foundation (dana.org), a non-profit organization that funds and disseminates brain research information, "Food-addicted individuals also have pre-frontal cortex (PFC) structural changes (for example, reduced volumes) which impede or impair the normal processing of the PFC." In other words, whereas a healthy PFC enables a person to clearly understand the painful consequences that lie ahead for poor decisions, a PFC altered by food addiction does not afford similar clarity about those consequences. Of the seven subcomponents that comprise the brain's reward center, this is the only one that tells the person, "No, don't do it; weigh the consequences." Therefore, it is easy to see how an impaired or altered PFC has a diminished capacity to carry out its original functionality; the "just say no" muscle is not fully functional.

In 2009 Dr. Gearhardt led a team at the Rudd Center for Food Policy and Obesity where they developed the Yale Food Addiction Scale. This is a subjective tool to measure the degree of food addiction. The scale's questions fall under specific categories that resemble the symptoms for substance dependence as stated in the Diagnostic and Statistical Manual of Mental Disorders. Dr. Gearhardt found that overweight participants who had higher food addiction scores showed different brain activity patterns than those with lower scores. Specifically in response to anticipating food, participants with higher scores showed greater activity in parts of the brain responsible for cravings, but less activity in the regions responsible for inhibiting urges during consumption.

Dr. Gearhardt also worked in conjunction with Drs. Stice and Spoor, fellows at the Oregon Research Institute, and documented that administration of sugar, fat, and flavor-enhanced foods to animals can result in brain changes and behavioral changes, such as withdrawal, that mirror the effects of substances like alcohol, heroin, and cocaine.

Why We Return to Our Old Eating Habits

Once we become addicted, any emotional imbalances will induce cravings for relief – in our case, food. These could be painful memories, being uncomfortable at a social function, seeing another food addict enjoying one of our forbidden foods, or watching a highly enticing food commercial. What addicts call "triggers" scientists refer to as "cues," or powerful emotional memories. Anna Rose Childress, M.D., a psychiatrist at the University of Pennsylvania, has used PET scans in studying relapse due to visual cues. During PET scans, radioactive elements are introduced into the brain to track cell processes, generating a three-dimensional image showing where the trace elements travel in the brain and how long they stay there.

Dr. Childress reports that drug-taking cues cause the brain to release a small spurt of dopamine: "This increase in dopamine feels similar to a small dose of the drug itself." Some people report they can even taste the drug in the back of their throats, though they haven't actually taken any. "They're having a miniature high before they even get there. It acts like a salty potato chip or the smell of the brownie across the room, the chocolate croissant in the window. It's a primer, it's a seductive pull." That small spurt of dopamine causes a craving for more.

Nora Volkow, M.D., performed brain scans on cocaine addicts while they watched two videos: one of nature scenes, the other of people using cocaine. She found that dopamine increased in response to the drug-taking scenes in proportion to the subjective reporting of craving by the addicts. This illustrates the power of cues and how they work unconsciously. Dr. Volkow says, "For these people, their lives and experiences have taught them that when they see others using cocaine, they're probably about to get rewarded with drugs too. So even though they consciously knew they weren't going to get cocaine, their brains had learned to expect the reward."

Cue-related relapse is tied to longer-lasting brain changes than were originally thought. For example, the hyperactivity of neurotransmitters associated with alcohol withdrawal can last as long as a year. Scientists suggest that relapse frequently happens because the spike in dopamine in the addict's brain is experienced in the "reward" system. When the food addict sees a delicious cue it overpowers the planning and decision-making portion of the brain, the prefrontal cortex.

As with all addicts, a food addict's motivation is biased to short-term pleasure. We have all experienced this phenomenon after months of exemplary dieting. We are overwhelmed by the short-term relief provided by a binge over the long-term benefits of staying on the diet. Enticing cues can rekindle the food addict's, cues operate swiftly and unconsciously, which explains why relapses happen so automatically. Many who've relapsed say they were "just having a taste."

Poor Dopamine Production

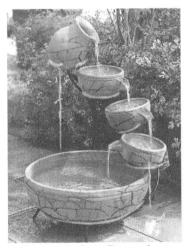

Figure 6 - Low Dopamine

What exactly caused the brain to become food addicted?

Let's take an in-depth look at what malfunctions in the dopamine generation process that fuels our overeating behavior. Using the previous cascading pots analogy, we see that if any of the pots are cracked, or if any of the supporting metal rings are damaged, the net amount of dopamine generated is compromised. A normal amount of dopamine is dependent upon the health of the entire infrastructure, starting with serotonin and culminates in dopamine.

The health of the genes responsible for the production of these neurotransmitters is vital to a normal level of dopamine. One analogy that I use to understand the importance of genes' health is a computer program, a set of instructions that is supposed to generate an accurate output. Some computer programs are very simple, for example they generate letters on a screen. Others are a tad more complicated, like one calculating the closing cost of a real estate purchase. Such a program accounts for multiple variables: commission to the real estate agents, pending taxes to the municipalities, administrative fees – you get the picture. If the code is faulty it will not generate accurate results in all cases. Likewise, any abnormalities in any of the genes necessary for the production of these neurotransmitters will result in a lower production of dopamine.

Flavor-Enhanced Foods

Until 100 years ago practically all of our food supply was unprocessed foods. We ate food that had a very short shelf-life, typically days, from the time it was picked or killed. However, our quest for convenience has led us to accept processed foods as our major source of nutrition. In most modern supermarkets one aisle is reserved for fresh produce in contrast to the 10 to 20 aisles of processed foods. Ingredients such as hydrogenated oils, high fructose corn syrup, and aspartame, to name just a few, have been proven to cause mild to severe disruption of our brain functions, but are readily accepted by most Americans. Our biology has simply not evolved to integrate all of these synthesized compounds at the rate at which they have been introduced. However, if you want to avoid highly processed foods you have to consciously plan your eating.

Today our ability to mass-produce food in the U.S. has generated an abundant and readily available food supply. However, experiencing pleasure with food was taken to a new level during the 1970s when the food industry began adding huge amounts of high fructose corn syrup, hydrogenated oils, salt, and flavor-enhancers such as monosodium glutamate (MSG). Between 1909 and 1999 sugar consumption per person nearly doubled in the United States. In that time, individuals went from consuming approximately 80 pounds of added sweeteners per year to 152 pounds – 64 pounds of which was high fructose corn syrup found in soda and processed foods. Scientists such as Robert Lustig, Ph.D., author of the book _Fat Chance,_ have taken on a crusade to make the American public aware of the biological changes that sugar causes. One of Dr. Lustig's findings is that overconsumption of sugar increases insulin secretion, which in turn blocks the generation of the hormone leptin. Leptin is the hormone used by the brain to manage the needs for more or less energy, so overproduction of insulin disrupts the chemistry of a healthy brain.

The massive amounts of sugar and prevalence of processed foods were just the beginning. The perfect storm ensued when the food industry took flavor-enhancing to the next level, as they discovered that these additives increase our pleasure and therefore their profits. This all occurred without most of us taking notice. The United States alone has thousands upon thousands of people whose sole job is flavor-enhancing. Flavor-enhancing was never questioned, and it has gained wide acceptance. Processed foods continue to be made tastier and tastier. Enhanced taste and large portions have become the American norm.

Our flavor-enhanced foods have recalibrated the sensitivity of our pleasure center. The brain develops a tolerance to the quantity and enhanced taste of the foods, which in turn rewires our brains to increase our dopamine level _only after_ consuming massive amounts of tasty foods. Unfortunately, that's not the worst news.

The really bad news is that we adapt to these large, tasty servings, and then we exhibit cravings more frequently than our Naturally Thin counterparts. Not only must we consume larger quantities just to avoid experiencing the blues or brain fog, but a study at the Obesity Prevention Center at Boston Children's Hospital documented that we are also compelled to eat more frequently. Once wired to overeat, the brain needs substantially larger amounts of tasty food to produce a normal amount of dopamine, and it needs them more frequently. Essentially the brain becomes a chemical thug. *"If you don't give me what I crave, I'm gonna make you feel really, really bad."*

Next, let's discuss why it is that certain foods have different effects on our hunger levels. The glycemic index was created to provide a measure of how quickly blood-glucose levels rise after eating a specific food. The food compound that has the quickest effect on blood glucose is pure glucose; hence it has the highest glycemic index, 100. The glycemic index estimates how much each gram of available carbohydrate (total carbohydrate minus fiber) raises a person's blood-glucose level. Most foods have been assigned a glycemic index value. Foods high in sugar have a high glycemic index; those low in sugar have a low glycemic index. When we consume anything with a high glycemic index we notice an immediate difference in how we feel. Foods low on the glycemic index, those low in sugar and carbs, must be converted to glucose by the body, so they have a very different effect on our blood-glucose level.

High-glycemic foods cause the release of the neurotransmitters dopamine and serotonin as well as enkephalins — endogenous opioids that make us "feel good." These neurotransmitters are also released with the use of nicotine, alcohol, cocaine, and heroin. Up to now many of us could not anticipate which foods would feel satisfying until our next meal and which foods would lead to overwhelming hunger a few hours after consumption. In June 2013, David Ludwig, M.D., Ph.D., Director of the Obesity Prevention Center at Boston Children's Hospital, found that consuming highly processed, rapidly digested carbohydrates can cause excess hunger and stimulate brain regions involved in reward and cravings. Using fMRI, the study showed that after a four-hour period following a "high-glycemic index" meal, the reward and craving centers lit up like a Christmas tree. This study is one of the first to substantiate what many of us experience as an overwhelming urge to eat even in the absence of physical hunger. This cycle is then followed by compulsive overeating of another high-glycemic index meal, which triggers dopamine euphoria, which then prompts another episode of intense hunger … it's a vicious cycle. Science has finally shown that continued overconsumption of sweeteners and highly processed foods can eventually change our brain chemistry and perpetuate cravings.

Foods high in fat and sugar are known to cause release of the natural feel-good chemicals known as opioids, which mask pain and promote euphoric sensations. Narcotic examples of these are heroin and morphine. When we eat Double Stuf Oreos,® the same brain receptors that respond to morphine and heroin respond to the neurotransmitters the cookies produce, just with slightly less pronounced effects.

Body Image

Over our history there have been changes in what defines a woman as sexually attractive. However, the most pronounced change happened in the late 1960s when attractiveness was redefined from curvy to androgynous. Because our biological imperative is to be attractive, for most women this fueled the never-ending compulsion to diet in order to achieve our tribe's new ideal of desirability.

Let's take a walk through history and examine what was considered attractive.

- In the 1800s, a large body was a sign of health and fertility. Corsets narrowed the waist and enhanced the bust.
- In the 1890s, actress Lillian Russell, at 200 pounds, was the most celebrated beauty of the era.
- In the 1910s, Paris designers created slim sheath dresses and declared that breasts were "out."
- The 1920s ushered in the era of the flat-chested, slim-hipped flapper, and the first dieting craze of the 20th century began.
- From the 1950s through the 1960s, the voluptuous full-figured shapes of Marilyn Monroe and Jayne Mansfield were celebrated.
- In the late 1960s, British model Twiggy, 5'6", around 91 pounds and size 0, arrived on the scene – and the diet industry exploded. In contrast, Marilyn Monroe who had been the icon of female sexuality was 5'5", weighed as much as 140 pounds, and reached a size 12.

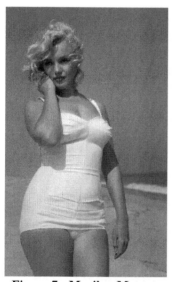

Figure 7 - Marilyn Monroe

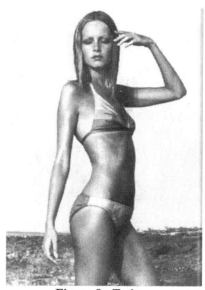

Figure 8 - Twiggy

- During the 1970s and 1980s, models gradually became taller, thinner and began to show toned muscle definition. Larger breasts made a fashion come-back.
- In the early 1990s, the waif-like figure of Kate Moss romanticized the wasted "heroin chic" look and a pre-teen body.
- The late 1990s brought in tall, very thin models with no visible body fat and muscles highly toned by hours of working out. Large breasts remained in style but were rare in this body type without the help of breast implants.
- Models in the 1970s weighed 8% less than the average woman; by the 1990s models weighed 23% less.
- Today the average American woman is 5'4" and weighs 160 pounds. In contrast, the average American model is 5'11" and weighs 117 pounds, or inch for inch, 34% less than the average woman.

Chronic Dieting

When we go on a diet in modern life, we attempt to lose our body fat by drastic reduction of food. This decrease then fires up the neural circuits, which deploy the army of hormones that trigger the imperative to overeat. We call these mechanisms famine brain for short. When we end the diet, the survival instinct fuels our overeating, preparing us to store enough fat for our next famine ... which for modern women will occur during our next diet.

Modern Lifestyle

Our frenetic lifestyle jumbles up the flow of our vital energy. There is no silence: we are connected via the radio, TV, Internet, and cell phone. Our brain is supposed to be plugged into something 24/7. Our modern lifestyle is one of über-responsibilities: children, mortgage, jobs, social commitments, house. We are also inundated by upsetting catastrophic events that we call the news.

The amount of physical exertion required by modern, sedentary lifestyles is orders of magnitude lower than in our days of hunting and gathering. In fact, for many of us it is challenging to schedule any exercise. We live without physical exertion in a body that is meant to plow fields or run marathons. The irony is that physical exertion is what contributes to our physical and emotional balance.

If your lifestyle makes you stressed-out, frazzled, and discombobulated, it is no wonder that anything that makes you feel calmer, even for a few minutes, is going to be overused.

What Next?

In June 2013 obesity was officially classified as a disease by the American Medical Association. In a statement released with the change in classification, Patrice Harris, M.D., a member of the association's board, said, "Recognizing obesity as a disease will help change the way the medical community tackles this complex issue that affects approximately one in three Americans." Dr. Harris suggested the new definition would help in the fight against Type 2 diabetes and heart disease, which are linked to obesity.

Scientists such as Dr. Volkow have documented the similarities between drug addicts and the chronic overeater. Dr. Volkow is one of the researchers ardently lobbying the American Psychiatric Association to classify obesity as a brain disorder that causes food addiction.

In 2011 Yale University created the Food Addiction Research Education task force, or FARE. According to its website, FARE "grew out of a commitment to share with the public the scientific community's increasing knowledge and understanding of how food affects the brain. FARE's founders realized that this growing scientific knowledge about food addiction was being hidden by the food industry itself. Much as we have learned that nicotine and smoking cause lung cancer, we are discovering that specific foods can be addictive and cause obesity." Beginning in 2011 a handful of the major food manufacturers (Post Foods, Kellogg's, and General Mills) voluntarily began to reduce the amount of sugar in children's cereals. Post Foods specifically announced that its children's cereals will contain no more than 10 grams of sugar per serving.

As we stated previously, Dr. Gearhardt developed the Yale Food Addiction Scale. This was the first subjective tool to measure the severity of an individual's food addiction. The Yale Food Addiction Scale has been scientifically validated and it is the tool we use to determine the level of your food addiction: SEVERE, MODERATE or MILD. Below is a user-friendly, abbreviated version of this assessment that can quickly measure whether you have a food addiction, and if so, to what extent.

The following statements can have responses of: Never, Once per month, 2-4 times per month, 2-3 times per week, or 4 or more times per week.

1) I find myself consuming certain foods even though I am no longer hungry.
2) I worry about cutting down on certain foods.
3) I feel sluggish or fatigued from overeating.
4) I have spent time dealing with negative feelings from overeating certain foods, instead of spending time in important activities such as time with family, friends, work, or recreation.
5) I have had physical withdrawal symptoms such as agitation and anxiety when I cut down on certain foods. (Do NOT include caffeinated drinks: coffee, tea, cola, energy drinks, etc.)
6) My behavior with respect to food and eating causes me significant distress.
7) Issues related to food and eating decrease my ability to function effectively (daily routine, job/school, social or family activities, health difficulties).

The following statements from the same food addiction assessment have Yes or No answers.

8) I kept consuming the same types or amounts of food despite significant emotional and/or physical problems related to my eating.
9) Eating the same amount of food does not reduce negative emotions or increase pleasurable feelings the way it used to.

The complete Yale Food Addiction Scale, its scoring, and interpretations of your level of food addiction can be found at our website, thinwomanbrain.com. Knowing your level of addiction is beneficial. A SEVERE level of food addiction typically requires some personal modification to the protocol to help you reach a MODERATE then MILD level. Please consult our website for these special cases.

The good news, and the reason for this book, is that we can rewire our brains and reverse the damage caused by chronic dieting and addiction to flavor-enhanced foods, through arresting the obsession and eradicating the behaviors that don't serve us: overeating and bingeing. While it is useful to understand what has led to our food-obsessed brain, what is life-enhancing will be restoring our healthy brain.

Chapter 3 Summary

In this chapter we review one of our key biological mandates: what wires us to survive. The imperative to overeat and store extra fat to avert any possibility of extinction due to famine is fundamental human physiology. Several factors have contributed to the astronomical growth of food addiction: radical sociological changes in body image, food enhanced to increase pleasure, chronic dieting, and a sedentary lifestyle. The biological response that was meant to ensure our survival has morphed into a trigger for compulsive overeating.

When we diet, we activate the famine mechanisms that were meant to keep us alive on fewer calories. These mechanisms also drive the imperative to eat whenever we have the opportunity. And because our tastier, flavor-enhanced food supply is now the norm, our brain generates less dopamine, which leads us to eat more in order to experience the pleasure we used to get with a smaller quantity of food. Our modern lifestyle has created *Homo convenious*: the modern woman who is wired to overeat. The scientific community has now shown that the cycle of overconsumption of flavor-enhanced food rewires our brains to be food-obsessed, and for many of us, that explains our chronic overeating. We experience famine brain as an overwhelming imperative to eat and eat and eat.

Learning that food addiction has a biological basis provided relief from the guilt and shame I felt for so many years of failed diets. OVEREATING IS NOT A PERSONALITY FLAW. OVEREATING IS NOT A FAILURE OF CHARACTER. Chronic cycles of dieting-craving-consuming highly processed foods rewire the brain to that of a food addict, altering our very thought processes and motivations. Understanding the process helped me gain the emotional acceptance necessary for lifelong mindful eating. It is astounding that these transformations have occurred in less than 100 years. Contrast that to how long it takes our biology to evolve, typically many thousands of years. Our external environment has changed, but the brain is still wired to react to scarcity and unpredictability; it is now wired to overeat at the slightest hormonal imbalance. None of these individual changes – the food supply, the change in body image, the chronic dieting, the modern lifestyle – is the single cause of our obesity epidemic. But combined they have led us to become the fattest nation on the planet. Overeating is highly associated with the top three killers in the United States: heart disease, stroke, and diabetes.

Scientists such as Dr. Nora Volkow, head of the National Institute of Drug Abuse, as well as many others, have documented the brain similarities between drug addicts and chronic overeaters. It explains the overwhelming imperative to eat. Luckily, we also possess the remarkable ability not only to recognize the food addiction mechanism, but also to eradicate it.

Introduction

Beyond the obesity storm there is a silver lining. Two scientific concepts, neuroplasticity and Cognitive Behavioral Therapy, are fundamental on our path to returning to a Naturally Thin Woman. Neuroplasticity is simply the ability of our brains to change throughout our lives. Despite long-held beliefs that after a certain age the brain was static or deteriorating, the science of neuroplasticity has demonstrated that you *can* teach an old dog new tricks! Cognitive behavioral therapy refers to a method of physically modifying the brain by consciously and deliberately altering our patterns of thought. Once we have consistently executed these alternate behaviors, changes in the brain can be measured using neuroimaging technologies.

Cognitive Behavioral Therapy

Cognitive Behavioral Therapy (CBT) was first developed by Jeffrey M. Schwartz, M.D., a UCLA psychiatrist, while working with patients with obsessive-compulsive disorder (OCD). CBT is based on the reality that our thoughts cause our emotions, which then drive our behaviors. To help you understand how CBT works, let's revisit Dr. Schwartz's major breakthrough.

The original group that Dr. Schwartz treated washed their hands compulsively. Dr. Schwartz first showed his OCD patients CAT scans of their normal brain activity. He then showed them photographs of dirty hands. The OCD patients would experience immediate anxiety, as measured by CAT scans. After seeing their before-and-after CAT scans and how their brains responded to the dirty-hand photographs, the patients were able to gradually change their automatic reactions.

Using mindfulness practices, Dr. Schwartz's revolutionary self-directed approach gradually rewired the OCD patients' brains to be able to view the dirty-hand photos without experiencing any anxiety. Encouraged by Dr. Schwartz's success, other medical and psychological professionals began exploring the applications of CBT beyond OCD. What follows is a brief survey of how CBT has been applied in other areas.

Michael Merzenich, Ph.D., a Johns Hopkins neurophysiologist, and Paula Tallal, Ph.D., a Cambridge University neuroscientist, worked with children with dyslexia and dramatically improved their reading accuracy when they were trained to distinguish between similar but distinct sounds. The success of these studies then led to the creation of Fast ForWord, an organization that has helped over 1 million dyslexic students in over 40 countries.

Edward Taub, Ph.D., a Columbia University neuroscientist, expanded the CBT protocol and developed constraint-induced movement therapy, which led to major breakthroughs in helping thousands recover from neurological injuries caused by stroke.

John Piacentini, Ph.D., another UCLA neuroscientist, has documented the effectiveness of CBT for Tourette's syndrome. Dr. Piacentini's CBT protocol includes tic-awareness training where the Tourette's patient is taught how to self-monitor for early signs that a tic is about to occur. Competing-response training teaches the patient how to engage in a voluntary behavior designed to be physically incompatible with the impending tic, thereby disrupting the cycle and decreasing the tics.

John D. Teasdale, Ph.D., an Oxford and Cambridge researcher, formulated his own CBT protocol for clinically depressed patients based on the multilevel theory of the mind called *Interacting Cognitive Subsystems* (ICS). The ICS model explains that the mind has multiple modes that are responsible for receiving and processing new information cognitively and emotionally. This theory associates an individual's vulnerability to depression with her reliance on one, and only one, of the modes available to her, which inadvertently blocks all her other options. Preventing relapse of depression is predicated on an individual's ability to disengage from the black-or-white thinking mode and to easily move among the many modes available.

At first there was difficulty in getting the scientific elite to believe that people could actually change how their brains work just by focusing their attention differently. This process was not only self-directed, but it did not include any mind-altering drugs or extensive psychoanalysis. Finally, after many and consistent successes, CBT is now internationally favored as a practical means of overcoming longstanding and disabling conditions, both psychological and physical. This positive, pragmatic treatment is now widely popular with therapists and patients alike. It involves the restoration of natural neural nets that change the way we feel about our compulsion – in this case, about food.

Yes, we food addicts have some faulty brain wiring that activates an overwhelming desire and enslaves us to eat when we are not physically hungry. However, what CBT offers is the ability to leverage the activity in the existing healthy circuits using mental focus. George Gilder, author of the book *Microcosm and Telecosm,* calls Dr. Schwartz's CBT "a daring rescue of the concept of the free will."

What the Heck is Mindfulness?

Let's examine the number one criterion for CBT to be successful: mindfulness.

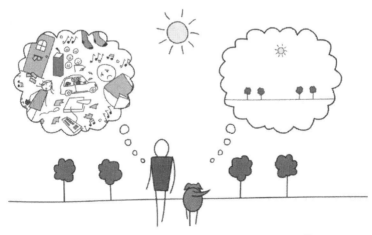

Mind Full, or Mindful?

Figure 9 - Mind Full or Mindful

The modern woman is typically not in the present; she is habitually re-examining past events and anticipating the future. Mindfulness means maintaining a moment-by-moment awareness of our thoughts, feelings, bodily sensations, and surrounding environment with acceptance and curiosity. It may not sound like a helpful thing to do; however, learning to experience the present moment in a way that suspends judgment and self-criticism can have an incredibly positive impact on our biology, our sense of well-being, and our ability to maintain equanimity during events that typically lead us to overeat. This then affords us a wider perspective, which leads to additional options and a sense of clarity when we execute decisions.

It's not just focusing on a teacher's lecture or a friend's conversation. It's "meta-awareness" – noticing where your attention is directed. So being mindful during a lecture means you are aware that you are paying attention. While driving, you don't just "keep your attention on the road," you are aware of the movements of your hands on the steering wheel, the motion of your neck as you check for traffic, the sounds of the road humming beneath you. Mindfulness is the ability to pay attention on purpose.

Mindfulness also requires acceptance, meaning that we pay attention to our thoughts and feelings without judging them – without believing, for instance, that there's a "right" or "wrong" way to think or feel in a given moment. When we practice mindfulness, our thoughts tune in to what we're sensing in the present moment rather than rehashing the past or imagining the future. It is intentional awareness.

In each moment, you are focused on the myriad aspects of the experience at hand. For example, when you serve dinner and your child immediately responds with, "But I hate chicken!!" you pay attention to your body's response, to the anger and frustration that bubble up. You notice the racing pulse, the "I worked so hard on this dinner after a long day…" You are not only aware of feeling anger, but also of accepting it, of accepting what is, without judgment. The following paragraph is how one of the leading mindfulness teachers, Jon Kabat-Zinn, described his progress.

"When I first started practicing mindfulness, I thought it was about seeing how everything in every moment was amazing and wonderful. One of the books I read suggested bringing mindful attention to washing the dishes, noticing the water, the soap, etc. So I tried it, and my inner monologue went something like this: 'Oh, the water feels so nice and warm, and that soap smells so good, and this feels so relaxing…' It was weird and bizarre, and felt mildly delusional. Bringing mindful attention simply means noticing and accepting what is. Noticing the sensations without ascribing a positive or negative value to them. Just noticing that there's water on your hands, or the scent of the soap. Noticing it, and not judging. No creepy narration as that's the left brain intruding. It is about being aware of our thinking, and responding in a balanced manner to challenges."

Bringing this type of mindful awareness to brain hunger is a relatively easy way to start your practice, as it should not involve a lot of emotion. And like acquiring any new skill, paying mindful attention to small occurrences of brain hunger will help you tackle the compelling desire to overeat. By being present we begin to weaken our overeating habits and disengage our unconscious responses. We also arrest the negative self-talk churning in our heads.

Most people find it helpful to know that there is a very high return on investment for their mindfulness practice. The easy analogy is developing physical muscles. When we hoist heavier and heavier weight, we alter the very fabric of our bodies in two ways:

- We increase our baseline strength.
- We increase our baseline flexibility.

When we invest in mindfulness, we practice formal procedures (one example is meditation) that alter the fabric of our consciousness in two ways:

- We increase our baseline clarity.
- We increase our baseline equanimity, the ability to remain calm even when faced with challenges.

The goal of weight training is not to achieve a temporary state of strength and flexibility that is present when you do the exercises and then vanishes during the rest of the day. The goal is to gradually increase your strength and flexibility. In other words, the purpose is to create permanent changes.

Similarly, the goal of your mindfulness practice is not to achieve a temporary state of clarity and equanimity that is present when you meditate and then vanishes during the rest of the day. The goal of mindfulness practice is to gradually increase your baseline of clarity, so that you immediately recognize what triggers your desire to overeat. Then you can calmly observe the overeating triggers with zero compulsion to act on them. It is not an intellectual understanding of overeating, but rather the ability to stay poised and confident, to simply observe your reaction to the overeating triggers.

As we begin to experience the benefits of equanimity, there is a ripple effect into every other area of our lives.

Leveraging Cognitive Behavioral Therapy

Earlier we presented some of the therapies based on neuroplasticity that have helped restore brain health to patients with a wide range of issues, including Tourette's syndrome, obsessive-compulsive behavior, depression, strokes, and dyslexia. Again, it is worth noting that via mindful observations (the ability to be in the present moment, including observing feelings and needs without judgment) we are able to modify the structure of our brains!

Clinical studies using before-and-after brain measurements have definitively quantified changes attributed to Cognitive Behavioral Therapy (CBT).

The question I had after learning about CBT was simple: can these types of therapies be leveraged to rewire our food-obsessed brains to not only reverse the damage that triggers famine brain but, *more importantly*, to help us adopt the behaviors of Naturally Thin Women? The answer was a resounding YES!

In Chapter 2 we explored the fundamental behavioral differences between Naturally Thin Women and those of us who are food obsessed. It is evident that if we could eradicate food obsession, compulsive eating, and mindless overeating, we could emancipate ourselves from the tyranny of diets. Rewiring the brain to have a healthy relationship with food bears no resemblance to Spartan self-discipline. Nor is it the anxious monitoring that allows so many women to stay *thin* but *stressed out*. Instead we reclaim the Naturally Thin behaviors as our automatic response to food.

Because your brain can change (neuroplasticity), the process of consciously repeating mindfulness practices will change the brain's neuronal circuitry at a physical level. You'll know you've reached a meaningful milestone when food no longer generates inner struggles that demand willpower.

In Chapter 2 we outlined nine distinct characteristics that are the hallmarks of a Naturally Thin Woman. Let's dig deeper into one of these key behaviors, specifically *eating only when we are hungry*.

First, to understand what physical hunger is, let's examine what is going on in the body. When our bodies have burned up the food in our stomachs and our blood-sugar and insulin levels begin to drop, the cells lining the stomach generate a hormone called ghrelin. Ghrelin communicates with the hypothalamus, which is housed in the deep center portion of our brain. The hypothalamus is what regulates our basic body functions such as hunger, thirst, sleep, and sex drive. Once it receives the message, delivered by ghrelin, that we need to eat something to keep our bodies running, the hypothalamus triggers the release of neuropeptide Y, which stimulates our appetites, producing tangible signs of physical hunger.

- Our stomach begins to grumble.
- There is a sense of low energy, perhaps queasiness.
- The taste buds on our tongue are fully awakened.
- We would welcome most nourishment; we are not *craving* a specific food.

In contrast, when we are wired to overeat, many of us will experience the *desire* to eat even when we are not physically hungry, typically in response to visual cues. This is called "external food sensitivity," also known as EFS.

Food addicts also respond to "situational hunger." Let's look at what situational hunger entails:

Social. Wanting to overeat to partake in a shared experience in the hopes that it will connect us to others. We tend to overeat, in a social setting, to avoid feelings of inadequacy or because we are not finding the party engaging.

Sensual. Eating because the food is there – at a restaurant, seeing an advertisement for a particular food, or passing by a fragrant bakery. The desire to eat is a learned reaction so tightly coupled with certain activities (such as watching TV, going to the movies, or attending a sporting event) that it becomes an automatic response.

Thoughts. Eating as a result of negative self-talk or making excuses for eating. The irony is that it can be triggered when we scold ourselves for lack of willpower.

Physiological. Eating in response to physical discomfort, such as headaches or other pain.

Emotional. Eating in response to stress, boredom, fatigue, tension, anger, anxiety, or loneliness. Instead of dealing with the underlying emotion in an effective manner, eating suppresses the emotion and shifts our focus to what initially appears to be pleasure; unfortunately after we eat, we then indulge in self-admonishment.

We can learn to observe the anxiety that situational hunger causes. Through my experience I developed the Thin Cognitive Behavior protocol (TCB), which is a specialized application of Cognitive Behavioral Therapy. It has four basic steps:

> Step 1: Recognize brain hunger
> Step 2: Observe the brain hunger
> Step 3: Name the real need and address it
> Step 4: Measure progress and experience success

The goal is to perform these steps consistently, for 21 to 42 consecutive days, until the rewiring is firmly established. The first three steps are especially important at the beginning of the process.

Step 1: Recognize Brain Hunger

Once we are wired to overeat, there are many situations and emotional imbalances that will trigger obsessive food fantasies and compulsive eating urges. Food craving has an actual physiological effect in our bodies. Our mouths start to water, and we produce dopamine just fantasizing about the pleasurable food. This can actually be measured as increased brain activity and heart rate. Our anxiety level rises; we *need* to experience that pleasure. The brain actually releases neurochemicals to lower blood-sugar content in anticipation of the upcoming sugar; that is why we feel shaky and cranky when we experience brain hunger.

The crucial first step is the ability to recognize brain hunger and name it for what it is. This is not accomplished by superficial, casual observation; rather, we mindfully gain awareness that the "hunger" that feels so compelling is not physical in nature, but rather an obsessive feeling, a compulsive urge. One useful aid is to review the signs of physical hunger (growling stomach, low energy, etc.) while taking deep breaths. The other is to ask ourselves when we last felt full. The process allows us to actively respond by telling ourselves, "This 'hunger' is not physical; this is brain hunger, this is a compulsive urge."

The goal of Step 1 is to assertively identify the brain hunger urge as a misfiring of the brain. Unequivocally, we must say to ourselves, "There is a biochemical imbalance in my brain. I'm currently wired to experience many situations and emotional imbalances as hunger."

This is not *resisting* the urge to overeat; we've already used plenty of willpower to stick to diets. Instead it is recognizing and naming the hunger for what it is without rattling our brains and creating additional anxiety. Learning to name brain hunger with calmness and clarity strengthens our ability to observe it without having to indulge in food. The willingness to recognize and accept that the hunger is not physical in nature is *huge* progress. Recognition is what halts the compulsive and automatic response to situational hunger; it changes the urge. However, it is important to remember that just recognizing situational hunger, without following through with Steps 2 and 3, won't diminish the hunger or make it go away.

Sometimes Step 1 causes anxiety, and if this is the case for you, we have dedicated the entirety of Chapter 5 to the practices available to develop mindfulness. Mindfulness is what will allow you to objectively observe brain hunger.

Step 2: Observe the Brain Hunger

The physical manifestation of brain hunger is real and tangible. Until recently scientists did not understand that the anticipation of pleasure itself generates dopamine in the reward centers of the brain. In the August 2012 publication of *Scientific American,* an article by Oxford's Morten L. Kringelback, Ph.D., and the University of Michigan's Kent C. Berridge, Ph.D., documented that the brain's hedonistic hotspots generate pleasurable feelings during food fantasies. Depending on the severity of the food addiction, once addicts start fantasizing about the rewards of eating, they experience not only pleasure, but also involuntary physical responses: they start salivating, their taste buds are sensitized, and they yearn for the sensual act of eating.

A significant number of neurotransmitters fuel this food trance. It grows and grows until we become zombie-like automatons. We enter into a vicious cycle of experiencing pleasure as we indulge the food fantasy until it overpowers us, and eating takes on a life of its own. That is why it is called an obsessive food-thought, and most addicts feel helpless under its grip.

Let's take a look at exactly what is occurring in the brain when we experience these food fantasies. As we outlined in Chapter 2, there are many chemical changes in our brains that have conditioned us for overeating. Chronic dieting has rewired our brains to experience famine brain even in the absence of food shortages. Biologically, we have an ability to experience pleasure from foods even when we are not hungry. We have come to believe that certain foods will meet our emotional needs for comfort, excitement, and relaxation, just to name a few.

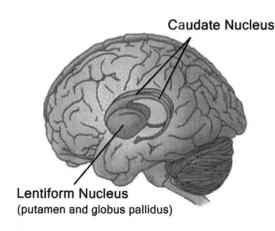

Caudate Nucleus

Lentiform Nucleus
(putamen and globus pallidus)

Figure 10 - Caudate Nucleus

Deep inside the brain lies a structure called the *caudate nucleus*. Scientists worldwide have studied this structure and believe that in people with compulsive behaviors, the caudate nucleus may be malfunctioning. Think of the caudate nucleus as a processing center for body movement, physical feelings, learning, and planning. Together with its sister structure, the *putamen*, the caudate nucleus functions like an automatic transmission in a car; they assure the smooth transition from one behavior to another.

During a normal day, we make many rapid shifts of behavior – smoothly, easily, and usually without thinking about them. It is the caudate nucleus and the putamen that make this possible. In compulsive persons, the problem seems to be that the smooth shifting of thoughts and behaviors is disrupted by a glitch in the caudate nucleus. As a result of this malfunction, the front of the brain becomes overactive and uses excessive energy. It's like having your car stuck in a ditch. You spin and spin and spin your wheels, but until you manually shift gears to get some traction, you won't be able to get out of the ditch. When compulsive overeaters get the "I'm hungry" feeling that won't go away, it's the same as spinning our tires. We have to switch from automatic to manual, from unconsciously accepting "I'm hungry" to mindfully exploring what is triggering the brain hunger.

There are several perspectives on how to interrupt these types of obsessive food thoughts. For those without any addiction, the overpowering force of the compulsion is a foreign concept. "What do you mean you couldn't help yourself? The food didn't jump in your mouth. Just say NO!" They simply don't get that when a rubber mallet hits the knee, no degree of willpower will stop that automatic reaction. That's why it is called a knee-jerk reaction. Duh! And as the ego depletion studies show, any strategy to subjugate food desire with willpower will not work consistently.

The University of Kentucky's Suzanne Segerstrom, Ph.D., postulated the theory that she called "Pause-and-Plan." Dr. Segerstrom documented that what we experience as an internal conflict is our inability to pause or slow down, and weigh the effect of "I want to experience that pleasure" versus "I shouldn't have that." This personal capacity is what determines our ability to execute an *interrupt step*.

When a food addict attempts to interrupt an automatic response to the craving with willpower, there is usually an emotional clash. In fact, the inability to use willpower can intensify the urge, taking on a life of its own and becoming a full-blown BINGE!

When he developed the original CBT protocol, Dr. Schwartz's brilliance was to measure that using willpower alone did *not* change the chemistry of the brain. Yes, Will-Powered Thin Women can derail what otherwise would be experienced as runaway food fantasies, but that is it! It is just suppression, and it requires hypervigilance every single day of their lives. More importantly, willpower doesn't change anything. Yes, it has been used many, many times as a short-term stop-gap, but it doesn't end the desire to overeat or the craving for food. And because willpower is a limited resource, we feel ashamed when we run out of it and succumb to overeating. Rewiring the brain is universes away from using willpower; it is the ability to observe the physical manifestation of food addiction calmly and compassionately!

Instead of attempting to override the food fantasy, the TCB protocol prescribes mindful observation of the physical symptoms – the salivating, the aroused taste buds, and the high anxiety. What this means is that we develop the ability to calmly and compassionately *observe* these physical manifestations without the compulsion to *act* on them. It is imperative to understand this distinction: Willpower is shouting to an unwelcome visitor to "LEAVE! GET OUT! YOU ARE NOT WELCOME!" Step 2 of the rewiring process is a different reaction: "Oh, hello, it's you again. I recognize you. I know what you want. I feel your power over me! I'm willing to acknowledge you, but I'm not going to indulge you."

Here is my analogy to crystalize this idea: I'm sure you have seen a child in a public place screaming at the top of her lungs demanding something from her mother by throwing a tantrum. There are three types of responses that the mother can exhibit: Acquiesce, Overpower, or Accept.

1. Acquiescing is when the exasperated mother gives in to the demands of the child because it's easier. She can end the agonizing embarrassment that the child is causing her.
2. Overpowering is when the mother starts yelling back and exerts her dominance to end the child's tantrum.
3. But on rare occasions, I have seen the mother lovingly kneel down by the little girl and acknowledge the child's demands, while informing her that no amount of screaming is going to get her what she wants. This is the nature of acceptance.

Acceptance is: I see your tantrum. I acknowledge what you want. I recognize your demands, yet I choose not to indulge them. No amount of screaming will shift me out of my equanimity.

In Step 1, we recognize the difference between brain hunger and physical hunger. In Step 2 we accept the brain hunger for what it is: our current wiring. During my rewiring, when I experienced involuntary salivating, I recognized it as a tangible manifestation of my food addiction. My taste buds were on fire, but I just accepted it as evidence of brain hunger. I accepted my fantasy of how good that ice cream/pizza/chocolate was going to taste! I didn't run away from it, I didn't try to ignore it, I accepted it compassionately for what it was: my food addiction.

Our ability to observe our addiction calmly, with compassion and acceptance is what rewires the brain.

Please Note: If you have a SEVERE level of food addiction and no mindfulness training, it might be necessary to lower the severity of your addiction before you are able to observe your brain hunger. On our website and in Chapter 6 we discuss tools that can be leveraged to short-circuit the food fantasies while your mindfulness abilities are developing.

Step 3: Name the Real Need and Address it

Depending on your personal triggers, Step 3 could be challenging. Our brains are constantly running programs, much as a computer does. We are aware of some of them; others are completely subconscious. Many of these programs are so ingrained that we have an involuntary response, akin to closing our eyes when we sneeze. The important point is to recognize that due to our current wiring, a variety of subconscious programs are fueling overeating.

By naming the need and addressing it, we stop the overeating and instead direct energy to what is currently masquerading as hunger. Some of the hunger reaction is due to situational triggers, but some might be due to habitual suppression of our basic emotional needs. If you have difficulty naming it, you might need outside help to get to the place where you are comfortable expressing your needs. For others it might require examining past history that could be causing you to repress the root issue. Are you stressed out because of work, money issues, difficulties with a loved one, etc.? Are you simply in a social situation where everyone else is eating and you unconsciously want to fit in? By naming the hidden need, you approach the process so that your emotions are not hijacked and you can address the true need instead of indulging in overeating.

Consistent repetition of Steps 1-3 changes the biochemistry of the brain and causes the atrophy of the neural nets that trigger situational hunger.

Step 4: Measure Progress and Experience Success!

Neuroplasticity (our ability to modify our own brains) occurs when we develop the ability to calmly observe brain hunger while experiencing zero anxiety. This doesn't happen overnight; like weight training, it requires repetition, which then leads to healthier wiring and breeds good habits. Practice reinforces the connections between the neurons (the cells that carry information in the brain) and makes them more likely to fire together in the future. A neural net essentially strengthens the affinity among neurons by reconfiguring their electrochemical relationship. The mantra of neuroscientists is, "Cells that fire together wire together."

Experiencing success generates a dose of dopamine. When we begin to feel good about our progress, it is indicative that the Naturally Thin Woman's neural nets are restoring themselves and rewiring is taking place. As we engage in more of the Naturally Thin Woman's behaviors, it should feel easier to generate some level of satisfaction. Remember that achieving goals also generates dopamine! When we don't experience success it means there's no acquisition of the Naturally Thin Woman's behaviors.

In my area of expertise, the computer industry, the importance of experiencing progress has been documented over and over again. In the famous paper "The Importance of Percent-Done Progress Indicators for Computer-Human Interfaces," the University of Toronto's Brad A. Myers, Ph.D., found that people prefer to have progress indicators while they are waiting for a task to complete. Software development teams where goals are 1) short-term, 2) shared with the group, and 3) where progress is prominently displayed are 90% more likely to successfully complete their project than those where progress is loosely tracked or not shared. In their book _Rules of Play_, the New School for Design's Katie Salen, Ph.D., and MIT's Eric Zimmerman, Ph.D., concluded that when the participants do not have a meaningful tool to measure progress, consistent engagement is unlikely.

We inherently feel good about achieving our goals, even when they are mini-goals. This progress increases satisfaction, which in turn increases the likelihood of continuing the rewiring process. In his article "Need to Complete," MIT's Hugo Liu, Ph.D., states "It turns out that when you finish a complex task, your brain releases massive quantities of endorphins."

Experiencing progress plays an important role in rewiring. It influences us to seek, complete, and comply with the Thin Cognitive Behavior protocol, which leads to successful long-term changes in our thinking. Without progress, there is no motivation. What has been proven effective is to tangibly track your progress in a manner that is meaningful to you, such as pasting an image on the front of the refrigerator that shows your weekly progress – in numbers, pictures and/or graphs. This could be progress in:

- recognizing non-physical/brain hunger
- recognizing your triggers

- effectively addressing what is fueling the brain hunger
- eating mindfully
- minimizing your external commitments (critical in avoiding "ego depletion") or
- managing your stress.

You are much more likely to complete the rewiring if you measure and genuinely experience progress as the rewiring occurs. Without motivation we will never complete the rewiring because there is nothing to keep us reaching for the next goal, the next improvement. We are more likely to give up when we can't acknowledge progress. Without motivation there is no progress. Without progress we don't complete!

"People often say that motivation doesn't last. Well, neither does bathing. That's why we recommend it daily." ~Zig Ziglar, author and speaker

Step 4 is where we assess the effectiveness of the TCB process; this is where we gauge whether our repetitions are paying off. When you experience brain hunger, simply compare this current situational hunger incident with its last occurrence. Ask yourself:

- After recognizing the hunger as situational, am I now able to identify the root cause of the misfire?
- Can I now effectively address the underlying trigger?
- In other words, how easy or difficult were Steps 1-3 this time? Were they effortless, flowing, and without trauma?

The psychological perspective of progress will inevitably shape our efforts and fuel our endeavors. This "Experience Success" step is where you rate your progress. Without any metrics, you are setting yourself up for failure.

I developed a scale to describe my personal levels of effort as I underwent the rewiring process. Please note, this is not a list for the sake of having a list. This type of scale is essential as we track our own progress. How the mind processes progress, as compared to stagnation, has a significantly different emotional payoff. Progress enhances endurance and boosts confidence.

If you find my scale helpful, use it. If not, I invite you to devise your own.

Subjective	Level of Difficulty
10	White-knuckle willpower, stratospheric anxiety, formidable concentration
9	Strenuous concentration necessary, extreme anxiety
8	High anxiety level, arduous concentration still required
7	Challenging anxiety, focus still required
6	Anxiety level still elevated and attention still necessary
5	Anxiety level still above normal, but manageable
4	Some anxiety, but high confidence that the step will be completed
3	Small amount of anxiety
2	Awareness of some anxiety
1	Zero struggle, zero anxiety

Because of the variety of issues and the range of complexity of situational-hunger triggers, this "Measure Progress" step will probably not score consistently for every single situational trigger. For example, you might find it easier to recognize progress in "needing a break" than in "feelings of inadequacy."

After using the TCB protocol, I understood that my "mid-morning hunger" was triggered by my inability to admit my physical limitations. Within a week of beginning the protocol, the intensity of "I need a snack" had substantially decreased to the point that I could immediately recognize this type of hunger as "I need a break." I could switch gears, take a walk, and return to work without any desire to snack. I measured my progress in the area of morning snacking, and it decreased from a 9 (strenuous concentration necessary) to a 2 (awareness of some anxiety).

On the other hand, dealing with a loved one, especially where there had been a long history of conflict, felt like spinning my wheels in the mud, and I measured zero progress. I simply got frustrated and ran to the refrigerator. I kept attempting to use the TCB protocol, but I could not get past Step 1 (I know that I'm not physically hungry). Finally, after recognizing that I was not getting anywhere, I admitted that I needed help in this area.

One of my friends suggested using active listening, a communication skill pioneered by Carl Rogers. In this process one person speaks and the second person has to reflect back what they heard before speaking themselves. This interaction is repeated until both people feel that they have been heard. Once I leveraged the active listening process, it took a full month of focused attention before there was any measurable drop in effort. It was gradual, but eventually it did reach a lower number. I have not resolved all my differences with this person, but now I am able to interact with her without resorting to overeating.

Notice that the first type of situational hunger (needing a break) boiled down to being able to address a personal need. However, the second type (conflict) entailed interaction with another human being. The second type necessitated additional resources (in the form of communication tools) before I was able to feel comfortable.

For this reason, it is important to discern between meaningful progress and recurring challenges. Little or no progress with a specific trigger typically means that this is an area where we need outside help. Going back to the car analogy, most of the time you can get out of the mud by shifting manually. However, if the mud is deep and gripping, you might need a tow truck.

On our website the personalized assessments provide situation-specific suggestions for areas where you find it difficult to make progress.

Mindful Eating

You certainly know this by now: Most Naturally Thin Women share several habits that result in a healthy relationship with food:

1. They eat only when they are physically hungry.
2. They invest the time to prepare healthy meals.
3. They focus on the eating experience; if possible they eat in silence.

4. They eat in a beautiful space.
5. They take pleasure in eating.
6. They take only small bites.
7. They frequently put their eating utensil down.
8. They chew slowly and thoroughly.
9. They consciously breathe before each bite.
10. They stop eating when the food loses its taste.

What is the foundation of most of these habits? *Mindful eating.* I was always fascinated when Naturally Thin Women used this phrase. Just what is mindful eating? I wanted to know exactly what they were doing when they ate mindfully.

In order to develop the habits of Naturally Thin Women, we are going to leverage the four TCB steps. Let's review them:

Step 1: Recognize the old pattern
Step 2: Observe the old pattern
Step 3: Mindfully execute the Naturally Thin Woman behavior
Step 4: Measure progress and experience success

Please Note: If your level of food addiction is SEVERE and you have no mindfulness training, it might be necessary to modify these steps before you are able to execute them. If you experience overwhelming anxiety in attempting these steps, please consult our website for "Mindful Eating Steps for Individuals with SEVERE Food Addiction."

Let's begin.

Habit #1 – Recognize physical hunger

Step 1: Recognize situational hunger – As discussed in Chapter 3 there are five types of *triggers* that initiate our current overeating programing. We are rephrasing them here:

Social Triggers: Wanting to eat to avoid feelings of inadequacy or to partake in a shared experience in the hopes that it will connect us. (There is scientific evidence that we eat substantially larger portions when we eat in a social setting.)

Sensual Triggers: Eating because the opportunity is there, for example: donuts at work or passing by a bakery. In these cases the desire to eat is a learned response to external triggers. We were not *hungry* until we experienced the *visual food cue.*

Thought Triggers: Eating as a result of an internal dialogue that is self-reproaching. We feel bad about ourselves, and the irony is that indulging the overeating behavior typically leads to scolding ourselves for lack of willpower.

Physiological Triggers: Eating in response to physical cues (for example, headaches or other pain).

Emotional Triggers: Eating in response to boredom, stress, fatigue, tension, depression, anger, anxiety, or loneliness. These triggers could be as simple as a lack of body awareness (I need a physical break) or as complex as repressed emotions (I am part of a toxic family).

Step 2: Observe the brain hunger – My brain is food-obsessed. I'm currently wired to experience hunger and respond compulsively toward food in response to a variety of situational triggers.

Step 3: Name the real need and address it – I have options on how I can effectively respond to the trigger depending on the situation:

Type of Trigger	Healthy Response
Social: I can taste a couple of tiny bites and rave about the food, so that I can achieve my desire to connect with others. Better yet, I can initiate an engaging conversation about something other than food.	This is not physical hunger. This is my desire to fit in.
Sensual: I recognize my habitual response to the visual stimulus of food. I admit that I was not hungry before I saw the food. I need to acknowledge that this is not physical hunger but an automatic response to an unexpected treat.	This is not physical hunger. It is my Pavlovian reaction to a highly charged stimulus, my desire to experience pleasure, and it reflects my deeply rooted belief that eating that treat is going to make me feel better.
Thought: I recognize my habitual response to negative thoughts, pain or discomfort; I want to get out of it; I want to end the emotional distress.	This is not physical hunger. I now have alternative and meaningful ways to address my feelings of inadequacy. Food is how I have habitually soothed myself and muffled my own painful thoughts. I possess the tools, or can engage the necessary help, to process the internal painful dialogue.
Physiological: Headaches, muscle and joint pain, or any other physical pain.	This is not physical hunger; it's a learned response to bodily discomfort. I have more effective tools (medication if needed) to cope with physical ailments.
Emotional: Sadness, anxiety, tiredness, anger, disappointment, etc.	This is not physical hunger; it is my default coping mechanism, my current wiring. I can identify what is triggering the emotional hunger and choose to address it in an effective manner. (Please refer to Appendix A for additional insights on this topic.)

Step 4: Measure the progress – After executing Steps 1 through 3, how are you feeling? The Subjective Level of Difficulty scale will help you gauge your progress as you adopt each habit. The more you practice, the easier it will become.

Are you able to appropriately respond to each trigger? If the answer is no, what is your stress level? Do you need to first lower your stress level? What are your meaningful choices to meet the actual need?

Habit #2 – Invest in preparing a healthy meal

There are so many benefits to home cooking:

- It is a form of mindfulness.

- You personally will select the high quality, nutritious ingredients. Remember that the food business is based on cheap fat and cheap carbs, not nutritional value to you.

- You regain control of where your calories come from: do they come from trans-fats, extra sugar?

- You ensure that there are no flavor enhancers, such as MSG and other brain-sabotaging ingredients. As previously discussed the net effect of these additives is that you eat more.

- Cooking a healthy meal is a form of expressing love to yourself and to your family.

- It is a creative outlet.

- It saves you money for activities like that exciting vacation to Tahiti, or Paris, or the Galapagos. ☺

- You can spend as much time or as little time as you want to invest. There are hundreds of online recipes for quick-and-easy meals. There are thousands of tricks and shortcuts to save time in the kitchen. It is just a matter of being honest and restoring your cooking skills.

- Going anywhere to pick up food takes time; get the facts straight, by the time you drive over there, park, get the food, eat it there or bring it home, believe me it takes longer than just stir-frying a healthy meal.

- And, drum roll please, you are safer than eating out. According to the Centers for Disease Control, over 22 million incidents of restaurant food-poisoning are reported per year due to bacteria, viruses, and parasites.

Think about it, you are committed to eating mindfully. The one area that affects 95% of that commitment is the quality of the food that you eat. Unless you know who is cooking the food and what ingredients they are using (cheap trans-fat oils? lots of sodium? extra sugar?), how can you actually take care of yourself?

Habit #3 – Sit down to beauty

Lay out a simple but beautiful setting, especially when you eat alone. No matter how *famished* you feel, take two or three minutes to make the setting appealing. If you feel that you don't have time, that you are in "too big of a hurry" and want to eat directly from the refrigerator, that is a BIG CLUE that you are obsessing about food and probably experiencing high anxiety.

Setting a lovely table might make you feel crazy until your Naturally Thin Woman neural net is restored. But remember, it is vital to calm yourself down before eating, as this is what heals the "famine brain." There are several options to reduce high anxiety levels: a few minutes of deep breathing, meditation, journaling, a brisk jog – whatever *you* find effective.

Remember to measure your progress: Were you able to set the table without any anxiety? If not, were you able to identify the source of your anxiety and take meaningful action to address it?

Habit #4 – Focus on the eating experience (if possible eat in silence)

In a culture that values multi-tasking, eating has been relegated to a side activity. We don't associate eating with nourishing our body. Eating is what we do mindlessly while we are engaged in more important tasks.

Have you ever automatically turned off the car radio while trying to find a new address? Instinctively we know that removing the audio stimulation sharpens our ability to focus on finding that address. Likewise, silence allows us to focus our attention on the food, to be completely present to the eating experience. Watching TV, interacting on the computer, speaking on the phone, reading a book, or any other activity is not a complement to mindful eating. In fact, it's a great way to overeat, as mindful eating requires undivided attention.

If there is any resistance to eating in silence, what will help the rewiring is to recognize that up to now we have eaten only when there is some other activity going on; it is a habit that we have developed over many years. Seldom is eating our primary focus.

Eating in silence allows us to *hear* the internal dialogue of how we are enjoying the food and the subtle messages from our bodies when we are satisfied. If turning off competing stimuli generates anxiety, then breathe and journal on what is causing the anxiety.

If you eat with your family, invite them to participate in the mindful eating process. Strive to turn off as many distracting devices as possible during family meals; it is an improvement over eating while multi-tasking. Share your experiences of the food. Eating slowly doesn't have to mean taking it to extremes. Still, it's a good idea to remind your family that eating is not a race. Encourage them to chew every morsel of food as they explore its tastes, textures, and smells in minute detail. Ask them about their own sensations, not to fish for compliments, but to value the blessings of sharing a meal.

Remember to measure your progress: After eating in silence, how are you feeling? Are you able to turn off all of the distractions and eat without any anxiety? As you practice this habit, is eating in silence getting easier?

Habit #5 – Take pleasure in eating

Naturally Thin Women have an internal dialogue of gratefulness, acknowledgment and pleasure: "This is really yummy," "Wow, I can taste the garlic, the basil, the sweetness, the lusciousness, the saltiness." This is the very dialogue that soothes and satiates the pleasure center of the brain. When we shovel our food, we not only miss out on tasting each morsel, but the pleasure center is not properly stimulated, so we need more food to meet our pleasure quotient.

Recognize that any resistance to this internal dialogue is the current habit of not being present to the pleasure of the food. Typically our dialogue has more to do with problems, worries, and "to-do lists," because we are feeding something other than our bodies.

When we can give 100% attention to the food and experience pleasure while eating mindfully, we have evidence that we are getting closer to restoring our Naturally Thin Woman wiring.

Remember to measure your progress: After allowing an internal dialogue that is about the joy of eating, how are you feeling? Are you able to experience pleasure in conducting this dialogue without any anxiety? If the answer is no, what are the obstacles to achieving this habit? Are you feeling foolish?

Habit #6 – Small bites

When we place too much food in our mouth, we consume more calories to experience the same amount of pleasure. We simply must recognize that we have a history of taking big bites. One meaningful action would be to eat a few meals with a tiny spoon, like training wheels, while we learn to take smaller bites. However, it's important to increase the size of the spoon once we have measured progress in this area. The reason is that if we take small bites only because of the smaller spoon, we are not restoring neural nets; we are wholly dependent on the tool. There is more information on the use of tools in Chapter 6.

Remember to measure your progress: After eating an entire meal taking only small bites, how are you feeling? What was your level of anxiety? Were you able to experience pleasure with such small bites? Did you have to run to the kitchen and get a larger spoon? Did you simply start eating with your fingers? ☺

Habit #7 – Fork down

Putting down the fork – or whatever the eating utensil is – between bites promotes mindful eating. We are poised to savor every bite, to experience every morsel, subtlety, spice and texture. Eating is not a race, it is foreplay. It is a sensual experience. Rushing through it defeats the purpose.

Remember to measure your progress: After eating an entire meal putting the fork down between bites, how are you feeling? How is your anxiety level? Were you able to taste the subtleties of the food?

Habit #8 – Chew slowly and thoroughly

For many compulsive eaters, a meal is the equivalent of a fix to a drug user. The faster they can shovel it in the faster they get high. Unfortunately, this behavior leads to a gross overconsumption of calories and shortens the pleasure sensation. We have a habit of trying to get our dopamine levels up as quickly as possible! Because we have done this for so long, when we attempt to slow down and chew mindfully, we are likely to become anxious.

Digestion begins with that first bite, which triggers the release of saliva, which in turn disinfects the food and lubricates the path to the stomach. While we are chewing, the brain releases the neurotransmitters that tell the hypothalamus that we are satiated. Chewing slowly and thoroughly also releases the subtle flavors and increases the pleasure of eating.

Remember to measure your progress: After chewing slowly, how are you feeling? How high was your anxiety level? Are you able to experience pleasure in slowing down without any anxiety?

Habit #9 – Breathing

Taking three breaths after swallowing reconnects us to our body; it is a type of palate cleansing, if you will. It recalibrates us for the sensual experience of the next bite. It's also a meaningful opportunity to gauge whether we are full.

Remember to measure your progress: Were you able to eat an entire meal where you took three breaths between bites? Did you experience any spike in your anxiety level? Were you able to experience pleasure in eating the food?

Habit #10 – Experience satiation

When we eat mindfully, we recognize that when food loses its taste, our body is telling us that it's full! In contrast, overeaters start looking for salt, ketchup, mayo, mustard, sugar, or barbeque sauce – anything that will restore a pleasurable experience and allow them to continue "*enjoying*" the food. The additives are an attempt to override the intelligence that signals you've had enough.

I'm sure you have heard the advice to wait 20 minutes to let your brain catch up with your stomach. By eating at the rate of a piranha, we consume massive amounts of food. We don't know how to wait, and by that time everything is gone. Besides, our brain is not that slow! We can immediately recognize when we are full if we are paying attention to when the food loses its initial appeal.

Be aware that when we begin this process it feels foreign. After all, we are used to consuming everything that's on the plate. For many of us, throwing food away is *mightily* difficult as our conditioning to eat everything on the plate is deeply ingrained. One helpful aid is to visualize the extra food as fat … in your least favorite body part. Your palate tells you when it has had enough, and any overconsumption will be turned into fat.

Also recognize that we are used to overstuffing our stomachs, so leaving food unconsumed might feel strange. At the beginning you will execute this step mechanically, but as you repeat it multiple times, you will experience genuine satiation. Moreover, restoring trust in your palate's signal is freeing, as you no longer have to experience feeling bloated after a meal. The satisfaction of having energy after a meal, instead of being lethargic and immobilized, restores your sense of freedom.

Remember to measure your progress: Were you able to say to yourself "That was great" and recognize "I'm full" without having to stuff yourself? Were you able to experience pleasure in recognizing fullness?

Chapter 4 Summary

Cognitive Behavioral Therapy (CBT) is one of the advances based on neuroplasticity that can help us restore our Naturally Thin Woman's brain. We have tailored this powerful technique into the Thin Cognitive Behavior protocol (TCB) to help us restore our Naturally Thin Woman neural nets. Our TCB protocol restores these neural nets in four steps:

> Step 1: Recognize brain hunger
> Step 2: Observe the brain hunger
> Step 3: Name the real need and address it
> Step 4: Measure your progress and experience success!

The power to rewire your brain lies in these four steps. These are the processes you need to succeed. Mindful eating, how a Naturally Thin Woman eats, can be broken down into ten basic habits:

1. Eat only when you are physically hungry.
2. Invest the time to prepare healthy meals.
3. Focus on the eating experience; if possible, eat in silence.
4. Eat in a beautiful space.
5. Take pleasure in eating.
6. Take only small bites.
7. Frequently put your eating utensil down.
8. Chew slowly and thoroughly.
9. Consciously breathe before each bite.
10. Stop eating when the food loses its taste.

Undeniably, much of our overweight society overeats and, in most cases, believes this is soothing and calming. Part of the TCB protocol is to relearn to eat "naturally," which means changing our current food-shoveling habits. The most profound change that allows us to eat for nourishment is to eat only in a calm, relaxed state of mind. It is not *eating the food* that calms us down, it is *eating in a relaxed state* that allows us to be properly nourished.

Learning to eat in a calm state of mind is a daunting task for most modern women. We are currently wired to believe that silence is boredom, that multi-tasking is efficiency, that investing in eating mindfully is a waste of time. Eating while under stress inevitably leads to overeating because all the mechanisms that allow us to eat mindfully are compromised. And conversely, eating mindfully also aids us in experiencing pleasure and recognizing satiation.

Naturally Thin Women exhibit most of the habits discussed in this chapter. By following the TCB protocol we begin to eat mindfully and to experience a great reduction of anxiety around food.

The next chapters will address some additional tools to ensure success in executing the TCB steps until we restore our Naturally Thin Woman neural nets. It's time to get down to the nuts and bolts.

Chapter 5 – Tools to Become Mindful

Mindfulness – Step 1: Recognizing Brain Hunger

As the developer of Cognitive Behavioral Therapy (CBT), Dr. Schwartz emphasized that recognizing and observing what is going on in our mind is THE critical ability in rewiring the brain. Again, the brain that can observe itself can change itself. Dr. Schwartz, borrowing from contemplative practices, referred to this ability as mindfulness: the state of being aware and present to the singular moment. And while the content of mindful experiences depends on our internal and external environments, mindfulness is usually characterized by a focused mind, a sense of being peaceful, and the ability to be keenly aware of our external world and the sensations in our bodies.

For the modern woman (*Homo convenious*) becoming mindful and gaining internal awareness might be the most challenging aspect of this program. But note that in order to execute Step 1, we need the ability to discern the difference between "brain hunger" and "physical hunger." When we are mindful, we have a minimum amount of anxiety, which helps us gain awareness of the internal dialogues that drive our overeating.

As stated previously, mindfulness develops from repeated practice, in much the same manner that consistent physical workouts develop muscles. And one way to develop your mindfulness muscles is through meditation.

As early as the 1970s, scientists such as Harvard's Herbert Benson, M.D., documented the many health benefits of meditation. More recently at the Medical University of South Carolina, an fMRI study headed by E. Baron Short, M.D., measuring the effect of meditation on brain functions, showed that just three hours of meditation led to improved attention and self-awareness. Julie Brefczynski-Lewis, Ph.D., and Antoine Lutz, Ph.D., at the University of Wisconsin documented differences between long-term and novice meditators. Specifically, for seasoned practitioners, disturbances (such as loud noises) had less effect on the brain areas involved in emotion and decision-making. The scientists documented that for people who had more than 40,000 hours of lifetime meditation practice (such as Tibetan monks), these areas were hardly affected at all.

Yet another study showed that after just 11 hours of meditation, researchers could measure changes in the brain. At UCLA, a study headed by Eileen Luders, Ph.D., focused on long-term meditation practitioners and documented a statistically significant increase in blood flow to the prefrontal cortex (PFC), which facilitates faster information processing. The PFC is the part of the brain that allows us to execute Step 2: Observe the Brain Hunger. More blood to that region indicates a higher ability to weigh the consequences of compulsive overeating.

Most studies show that meditation leads to mindfulness and positively affects not only the brain, but the whole body. A partial list of benefits includes:

- Lowering blood pressure
- Promoting the relaxation response
- Increasing energy level
- Improving the ability to sleep

- Improving the quality of sleep
- Lowering stress level, and
- Improving mental acuity.

Any of these benefits all by itself would contribute to a higher quality of life. But in our quest to restore our Naturally Thin Woman neural nets, meditation is the single most effective practice to help us achieve that goal.

In recent decades, research on meditation has grown substantially, in part because of the support of high-profile leaders like the Dalai Lama. Specifically, what scientists are finding is that meditation harmonizes the brain subsystems that are responsible for awareness: awareness of our physical body in space and awareness of what is going on inside our body. Body awareness is one of the factors that help us to differentiate between being comfortably satiated versus feeling bloated or stuffed.

Modern life is stressful by nature. When we are stressed out, our entire biology is focused on supporting the fight-or-flight response, leaving fewer resources for maintaining mindfulness. Consequently, if we try to dive into mindful eating while our bodies are producing high levels of fight-or-flight hormones, we will probably find the experience counterproductive, which will contribute to an even higher level of stress.

Eating mindfully is not a mechanical process; we can't just run down a checklist. I'll bet all the tea in China that attempting to robotically execute these steps will dramatically raise your anxiety level. And why is that? The mindfulness that we are striving to achieve is effortless and calm and is a result of the practice of slowing down and quieting our minds. Most people find it extremely challenging to throttle down overnight from the frenzy of modern living to a state of mindfulness.

Until I began a daily mindfulness practice, my ability to eat in a calm and relaxed state was simply not realistic. No amount of information was going to change my biology. Instead of fretting about what I should be eating, I began to trust that my meditation practice would be the lighthouse to guide me back to restoring my Naturally Thin Woman neural nets. I was able to turn the corner after only a few weeks of meditation, and then I began to eat like a Naturally Thin Woman. By investing in mindfulness practice, everything else fell into place.

The Most Documented Mindfulness Practice

Scores of university studies, leveraging the dramatic advances in brain-imaging technologies, have documented the value of meditation. Scientific papers have presented evidence that regular meditation increases efficiency, sharpens mental acuity, boosts our productivity, improves quality of sleep, and stimulates creativity. According to a study, headed by T. Wang Kjær at the John F. Kennedy Institute, consistent meditation practice can increase dopamine production by 65%! These are amazing bonuses, but for our purposes, what is most important is to understand that meditation fosters the restoration of the Naturally Thin Woman's neural nets.

During meditation, the areas of the brain usually involved in verbal thinking become quiet, and completely different areas light up. Our ego dissolves and we feel connected with the entire universe. This phenomenon is brilliantly illustrated by Jill Bolte Taylor, Ph.D., a Harvard-trained neuroscientist who suffered a massive stroke in the left hemisphere of her brain. For Taylor, the stroke was a blessing and a revelation, which she recounts in her book *My Stroke of Insight*. She shares that by "stepping to the right," away from the left side of our brains, we can uncover feelings of well-being that are often sidelined by "brain chatter." Dr. Taylor's book is an emotionally stirring testimony that inner peace is truly accessible to anyone.

What has been repeatedly described by contemplatives is that meditation is where the outside world becomes a quiet background and where we can meet the Beloved, which can be interpreted as the true Self. Despite all the evidence that meditation is the one practice that would dramatically increase our ability to eat more mindfully, people typically argue that they don't have time to fit it into their busy lives. We have lost the ability to determine which goals really matter. We have ceased to be human beings and have become human doings. We share a powerful collective resistance to meditation and seem to feel more virtuous the busier our lives are.

The average white-collar worker receives 300 messages per day via cell, text, email, faxes, Skype, WebEx, you name it. Our society has come to believe that we can solve our stress by finding the right gadgets. We search for devices that allow for speed and efficiency as we continue to plummet toward burnout. For many of us, the challenge in starting a meditation practice is that being by ourselves is unsettling. We stay in marriages where we can't grow because of our fears of being alone. We perpetuate jobs not aligned with our passions because of our fear of being outside the tribe.

Through meditation, we can reach a point of perfect stillness at the center of our being, a purity that is beyond what can be accessed by our five senses. From this core, this infinitely fertile emptiness, springs all that is authentic about us: our identity, our ability to recognize truth, that small voice that provides guidance, the absolute peace within our own genuine Self. Tapping into this infinite core is the *key* element of Step 1.

I was intrigued by the Grand Canyon-sized gap between "I'm interested in doing anything that would help me lose weight" and the excuse of "I don't have time to meditate." There is a cognitive dissonance between a society that says *busy* is good and the science that definitively proves that mindfulness is what would make a profound positive difference in our lives. What I now understand is that our ability to maintain a meditation practice is predicated on other factors:

1. The capacity to be by ourselves in silence. Initially, for most people there will be a period of anxiety. For me, there was one session where I felt like cockroaches were running on my body. My inability to sit with my silence was intolerable. But like a wound that begins to itch as it heals, this is a sign of progress.
2. Resolution of past trauma – childhood traumas top most people's lists.
3. Healthy relationships, or at a minimum the recognition of unhealthy ones.
4. The willingness to look at anything that no longer serves us.

When we start a meditation practice many of us might only be able to sit for 5 minutes as our anxiety level might be stratospheric. But once we start, we can gradually increase the time to 6, 7, or 10 minutes and eventually sit for 15 minutes, ideally twice a day. At the onset people have different tolerances, but gradual progression is what leads to success in restoring Naturally Thin Woman neural nets.

Active meditation – Every method of meditation is organic to an individual situation, to a unique mind, to a particular woman. Methods devised thousands of years ago might not be effective for you, the modern woman. For many of us, when we have not yet resolved our inner pain, it may be unbearable to pursue a *sitting* meditation practice. The moment we attempt to still our bodies, we may experience the monster of unprocessed grief or fear yammering at the door of our unconscious mind. This can trigger an intense fight-or-flight reaction, flooding our bodies with adrenaline that renders us angry, anxious, or restless, rather than peaceful. There are other forms of meditation that are active and might be better suited to fit those needs.

If you find that traditional meditation absolutely doesn't work for you, it doesn't mean that no method is useful. It only means that what is useful for me may not be useful for you; the methods themselves must be tailored to your individual needs. Any active meditation that does not generate an adrenaline surge will be a better option for people for whom sitting feels agonizing. Examples of mindful movement range from Dynamic or Kundalini meditation to rollerblading, long walks, yoga, jogging, swimming or T'ai Chi … any movement that you can conduct for at least 15 minutes where you stop making lists, worrying about the past, or thinking about the future. Anything that allows you to be 100% in your body, without the chatter of the left brain, develops mindfulness.

Other Practices to Develop Mindfulness

PQ Reps – Shirzad Chamine is a Stanford Ph.D. and chairman of the largest coaching-training organization in the world. Dr. Chamine works primarily with senior executives and lectures around the world about the profitability of mindfulness as a powerful tool to become more effective and build proficient teams. In his book, *Positive Intelligence,* Dr. Chamine discusses developing mindfulness by becoming aware of our bodies and environment for 30 seconds 100 times each day. Chamine labels these hyper-awareness moments as Positive Intelligence Quotient repetitions or PQ reps. For people who are resistant to sitting for any length of time or active meditation, PQ reps might be more feasible. They are akin to toning a muscle by executing lighter but more frequent repetitions.

Conscious Breathing – Many people are aware that, in physics, matter and energy are considered to be different manifestations of the same thing. One way to look at the body-mind connection is as a cloud of energy, where breathing is the bridge between the two. Through conscious breathing, we interrupt the chattering "monkey mind" and reconnect to our bodies.

Breathing diaphragmatically *into the belly* and feeling the torso expand spherically as you inhale characterizes conscious breathing. The *quality* of awareness (the focus and feelings evoked as we breathe) fosters mindfulness. When inhaling deliberately we transform regular breathing into conscious breathing, the kind of breathing that reconnects us to our bodies and brings us into the present moment. Awareness is what neuroscientists identify as the first step of the CBT protocol. The more we are connected to our bodies, the more likely we are to succeed at the Thin Cognitive Behavior protocol.

Mindfulness Aids

Some examples of alternative aids that if done frequently (100 times a day) could foster mindfulness are:

Smiling in public – Not only will you feel better just for smiling, but when you engage someone, there's a positive energy exchange.

Naming your mood – The same activity done in different moods will yield different results. Become aware of how your mood affects your biology.

Reconnecting with your body – Notice the position of your body and how that affects you. Is your body tense, or is it open and fluid?

"Returning to yourself" before being with another – Before engaging another human being, whether in person, by phone, or by email, breathe and return to yourself. When the phone rings, it becomes a reminder to re-engage in mindfulness. The person who is calling gets a *fresh* you, present and available.

Something old, something new – When walking along a frequently taken path, strive to notice something new: the chirping of birds, the slight drone of a plane overhead, or the sound of your own steps.

Indulging the child within – It could be as simple as lying on the grass. At first you may feel foolish, but don't let others' opinions rule your life; just feel the blades of grass, the breeze, and the sun on your skin. When I treat myself to this simple pleasure, it always brings me back into the moment and gives me a sense of childlike wonder that lasts the rest of the day.

Choosing to go slowly – It is a quality that reconnects us to the eternity of the present moment.

Within each of these moments of awareness we return to *the power of now*, which is also the title of Eckhart Tolle's phenomenally successful book. Tolle awakens his readers to their egocentric lives as creators of suffering and invites them to enjoy a pain-free existence by living fully in the present. This book is highly recommended for anyone interested in acquiring Naturally Thin Woman behaviors through the power of mindfulness.

Mindfulness Triggers

Remember that the TCB protocol is predicated on awareness of the present and feeling connected to our bodies. Mindfulness triggers are powerful tools to snap us out of "automatic pilot," the left brain chatter. Then we can return to a level of awareness that allows us to interrupt unconscious patterns. We can let go of past and future, which releases any emotional turmoil.

Mindfulness triggers can also originate with everyday activities or objects. Below are examples:

1. The Buddhist teacher Thich Nhat Hanh suggests posting little notes that will remind you to smile and relax. Notes that we can see first thing in the morning set the tone for the day.
2. We can download Zen chimes that remind us throughout the day to detach from the flow of habitual emotions and mindfully reconnect to our bodies.
3. Many people find that "transitional events" are the most useful mindfulness triggers. When we walk through a door we recognize that one thing is ending and another is beginning. We can say to ourselves, "I'm opening my heart; I'm reconnecting to my body before engaging in my next activity."

If we are in the habit of being mindless, we move from one experience to the next without that "emotional palate cleanser." What exactly is it that allows us to return to the present? The point is to always be in our bodies, not in our monkey minds (the restless, unpredictable, uncontrollable way that we swing from one thought to another). Mindfulness triggers are aids that provide us with "wake-up calls."

Interruptions are inherently stressful. When we pause before we migrate into another activity, it reminds us that we have choices. We can choose to calm ourselves by consciously taking a few deep breaths, which allows us to continue in a poised and gracious state of mind.

Getting Started

Rewiring begins when we can recognize the early warning signs of the compulsion. Some people call this being fully present in the moment, being mindful, or becoming the observer. Without this ability, we experience our craving as an overwhelming need to shovel a specific food into our mouths as rapidly as humanly possible. Without mindfulness, we lack the ability to step back and observe the tornado without becoming engulfed by it.

When we are able to *recognize* the compulsion, then we can *tell* ourselves: "Ah, all those nasty chemicals are tweaking my brain. I am currently wired to be a food addict, and my brain is executing its *overeating* program." This is Step 1, recognizing the brain hunger and naming it for what it is.

If you want to establish a solid foundation, one option is a meditation retreat. If you live in a big city and can find an organization offering meditation, you might invest in multiple sessions over one weekend. If you have the discipline to sit on your own at home, even if it is just 15-minute sessions Friday after work, Saturday morning and afternoon, and three on Sunday, you will be well on your way.

However, if the mere word meditation stresses you out, try one of the other forms of mindfulness practice. If a silent 30-minute power walk where you keep returning to your breath helps you get started, that is great! Just remember that every time your mind wanders, return to your breath as you continue your power walk. Please note that this is a *silent* power walk, no iTunes or iPhone, just an iLoveMyself mantra.

Another option is joyous, aerobic movement such as dancing. These activities replace the dopamine boost that used to come from sugar-laced binge foods. Exercise has the added benefit of reducing cravings and easing depression.

The ability to remain in the eye of the storm as you watch the tornado whirling around you is how we rewire our brains. Once you experience self-observation, you can invoke this new skill every time your old wiring wants to hijack you into an overeating frenzy.

Challenges to the Rewiring Process

The biggest challenge will be the departure from mainstream values such as multitasking (the antithesis of being in the moment). Typically we are in a hurry, obsessing about our next goal, completely disconnected from our bodies. Activities that might be soothing and healthy to our nervous system are often labeled *mindless*, an indication of how our culture gives no value to non-intellectual pursuits. Our thinking brain is in charge. We do not live mindfully.

Minimizing those activities that add more stress to our lives will demand a lot of courage. We must joyfully embrace our humanity, our need to love and be loved, our need for fun, sensuality, and creativity. When we live mindfully, we can stop committing to things that don't contribute to our joy.

We will have to recognize lies like "I don't have the time," "I don't have the energy," and "I don't have the support." The truth is we lack the COURAGE to live a life that nourishes us, and most times it appears easier to get that nourishment from food.

What if we were filled with mindfulness instead of food? Then we would be able face day-to-day challenges and disappointments with equanimity and peace. Have the courage to say YES to a higher quality of life.

Training Wheels and Stepping Stones

Google "eating mindfully" and you will find over 100 products (examples are mindful chimes, mindful eating cards) supporting that objective. While some of these products might be helpful, it's important to differentiate between mechanically using aids and restoring neural nets. When the only way to carry out a skill is relying on a specific aid, we are not restoring neural nets, we are merely relying on a crutch.

Think about this analogy. Training wheels on a bicycle are very helpful because they engage only if you start to tip over. They let you develop the balance required to ride a bicycle without getting in your way. Slowly you experience longer and longer periods where the training wheels don't touch the ground. Then one day you are so confident of your newly acquired skill that you take the training wheels off.

In contrast, a life vest is an invaluable aid if you find yourself in rough waters, such as river rapids or an ocean storm. But imagine using a bulky vest during swimming lessons in a shallow pool. Wrong! The life vest then becomes a deterrent to acquiring the ability to swim. You might learn to paddle around, but you will never truly master swimming.

If you rely on products to help you "eat mindfully," it is like learning how to swim while wearing a bulky life vest. Neural nets are not restored by using crutches and gadgets, though some of them are helpful if used in the initial stages. But if they come to be relied upon, the aids are in fact keeping you from restoring your neural nets. The danger is that once those aids aren't available, you may revert back to old behaviors.

Any products that you use to improve mindfulness must be used as stepping stones, helpful to guide your path. But if you are not experiencing progress as you decrease their use, you are not forging a path toward a healthier you. Training wheels are only for beginners; once we develop the sought-after skill, they must come off.

Chapter 5 Summary

Recognizing brain hunger is the first step of the rewiring process. Attempting to rewire when our anxiety level is stratospheric only compounds the problem. A mindfulness practice affords us the equanimity to become physically aware of our bodies, to readily accept our emotions, and to buffer ourselves from unhealthy reactions. When we are mindful, we are able to recognize a craving (whether due to an awkward social setting, peer pressure, or feelings of inadequacy) and engage in alternative practices instead of helplessly indulging in overeating.

The tool most widely reported as helpful to achieve mindfulness is meditation. If the thought of meditation freaks you out (and that's understandable for today's modern woman) try a form of *active* meditation (such as swimming).

There are other helpful tools for arriving at mindfulness: choose to focus on breathing several times a day, move through life at a slower pace, or become more aware of your surroundings (try noticing something new every hour).

What is critical is *choosing to become mindful*. It doesn't just happen on its own. Developing mindful triggers, like the ones listed in this chapter, can help remind us to live an aware life. Remember, we must be mindful to recognize brain hunger and what is really asking for attention. You'll know your neural nets have been restored when you can experience a food panic, calmly watch yourself name it as brain hunger, and identify which emotional need must be addressed. This is an experience with little struggle, minimum anxiety, and no compulsion to overeat. It is transformational.

Chapter 6 – Pattern Interruption
Tools for Step 2: Observe the Addiction

Many of us have experienced computer slow-down. We discover that, unbeknownst to us, there is a Trojan or rogue program that has installed itself and is consuming our computer's resources. Your current wiring is like those Trojan or rogue programs. It is time to delete them and stop them from misappropriating your mental resources.

Hopefully by now you understand that, due to chronic dieting, your brain is food-obsessed; you are currently wired to overeat. Passing by a bakery will trigger an overwhelming desire to taste that warm bread. Experiencing a high level of stress will have you eating directly from the refrigerator. Donuts at the office will trigger the program, "but so-and-so will feel offended if I don't appreciate her gesture." Any temptation will initiate the Trojan program called "Food Hypnosis!" Let's examine what is going on in the brain of the food addict.

As we shared in Chapter 3, once the addict starts fantasizing about food, the brain generates dopamine. Food fantasies trigger involuntary physical responses: we start salivating, the taste buds are sensitized, we are primed for eating pleasure. What is fascinating is that the fantasizing experience can generate even higher amounts of dopamine than actually eating the food. It's not only the act of eating that generates pleasure. For a food addict, the food fantasy creates a craving that is almost impossible to ignore. It overwhelms any ability to weigh the pros and cons of that desire. In fact, inside the brain, the part that allows us to switch from one activity or thought to another is stuck, like tires spinning in the mud. At the same time, the part of the brain that weighs the pros and cons of any decision is negatively affected. The vision of pleasure is not only compelling psychologically, it also triggers overpowering physiological reactions that lead to what is described as an automatic eating response.

Scientists have validated what many food addicts constantly wrestle with: our desire to eat in the absence of true physical hunger is overwhelming. In Step 2, we mindfully witness all of these bodily sensations and accept them for what they are: our current wiring. On top of all of these physiological sensations, *we believe that satisfying that food fantasy is going to make us feel better.* But it is just the opposite; the fact is, we feel ashamed after the indulgence. The addiction is to the cycle of shame. And unlike with other drugs, the physical effects of food addiction are evident to everyone around us – we can't hide being fat.

In Step 2, we recognize the physical sensations of the food fantasy: the pleasure we experience in anticipation of eating. Please note (and this is an important distinction): what restores a healthy brain is not suppressing these desires, not ignoring these physical responses, not distracting ourselves with something else. What helps us to rewire is the serenity and sense of accomplishment as we observe the manifestations of our addiction, which in the past would have led to an overpowering emotional undertow.

Understanding how to *build* muscles does not *develop* muscles. Similarly, understanding addictive mechanisms will not automatically allow us to observe our own compulsion. Our ability to just observe is a function of our mindfulness practice (see Chapter 5), which is why without acquiring mindfulness, food fantasies overwhelm us. Naturally Thin Women do not experience these powerful food fantasies; they do not have these types of automatic physical responses. They do experience physical hunger, but they do not experience the additional physiological changes that overwhelm a food addict. Naturally Thin Women's brains function differently!

When we begin to challenge our long-held belief that indulging our fantasies will bring us pleasure, it feels foreign. However, as we develop the ability to observe ourselves and to face the truth, the process becomes easier. Acquiring this ability is progress! When faced with food fantasies, take a few minutes to do deep breathing or journaling until you can recognize that, once again, you are being conned.

While you are developing the mindfulness muscle, and especially when the food addiction level is SEVERE, we are providing you with a couple of techniques that should be helpful in interrupting the food fantasies.

Eye Movement Desensitization and Reprocessing

Widely known as EMDR, this technique was originally documented by Francine Shapiro, Ph.D., in 1987. EMDR explains that our eye movements are intimately intertwined with our brain processes. So when we are recalling how delicious that pie à la mode *tasted*, our eyes automatically look up and to the left. When we salivate merely thinking how wonderful it is *going* to taste we look down and to the right. The graphic in Figure 11 depicts how our eyes move to the left when we are *remembering* food and to the right when we are *fantasizing* about food. Depending on whether we are fantasizing, hearing, or remembering, our eyes will move up, sideways, or down.

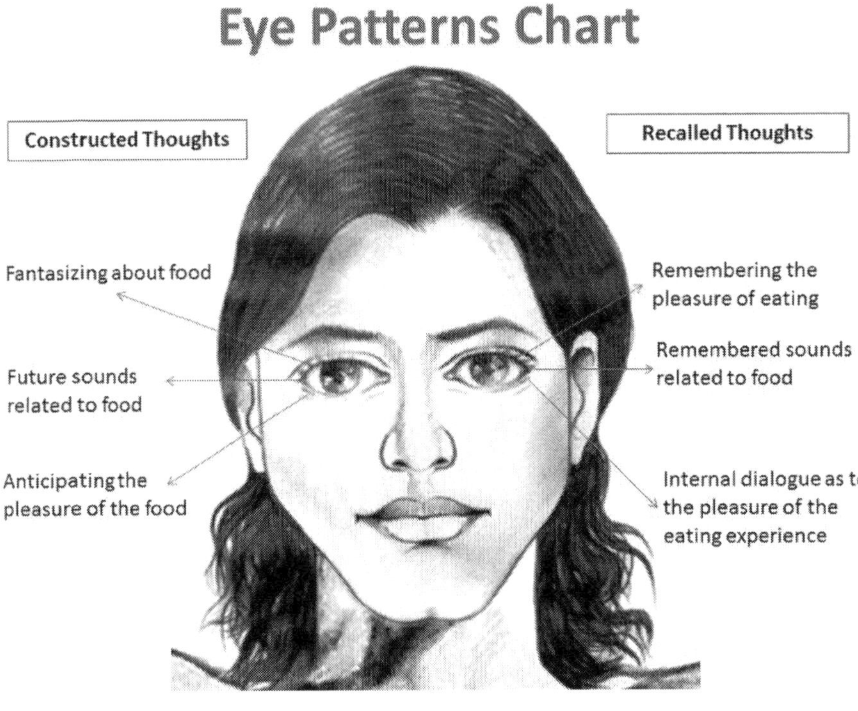

Eye Patterns Chart

Constructed Thoughts

Recalled Thoughts

Fantasizing about food

Remembering the pleasure of eating

Future sounds related to food

Remembered sounds related to food

Anticipating the pleasure of the food

Internal dialogue as to the pleasure of the eating experience

Figure 11 - EMDR Patterns

The importance of adding EMDR to our toolbox is that when we catch ourselves fantasizing about food (looking up and to the right), we can interrupt the pattern by rapidly moving our eyes in all directions until the craving stops. EMDR is a simple, easy, and effective tool that requires only 30 seconds of rapid eye movement to shift our brains away from obsessing about food. This interruption mechanism provides us the ability to halt the undertow when the food fantasy starts pulling us in.

Emotional Freedom Technique

Also known as EFT, this is another tool that has proven helpful for pattern interruption. The acupressure points were identified by the Chinese centuries ago as the ends of energy meridians in the body. When pressure is applied to these points we shift the energy in our bodies.

The EFT process uses your fingertips to tap these acupressure points rapidly until the emotional energy shifts. The points used in EFT are shown in Figure 12.

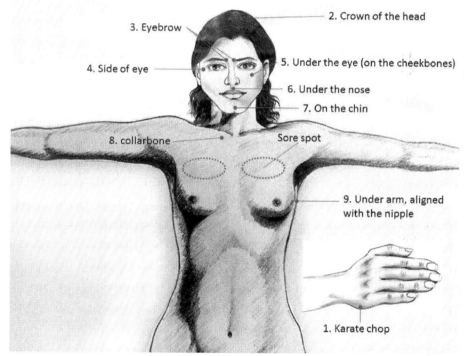

Figure 12 - EFT Pressure Points

If you want to learn the EFT process, there are hundreds of YouTube videos that you can watch.

First, ask yourself on a scale from 1 to 10, where 1 is none and 10 is overwhelming, how strongly you are experiencing brain hunger. Let's assume that you are at a 10. You start by tapping on the karate chop point while repeating the following set-up statement three times:

"Even though I'm experiencing overwhelming brain hunger, I deeply and completely accept myself."

EFT only works if you *believe* your set-up statement. If you say the statement out loud and you feel that it is not true, then you need to modify your statement to be congruent with your belief. For example, you might change the set-up statement to something like:

"Even though I'm experiencing overwhelming brain hunger, I believe that with practice, I can change my automatic responses."

Then begin tapping through the rest of the points, starting with point 2 at the crown of the head. While you are tapping, express your feelings. You might say: "I'm sick of this. When will this end? I'm feeling frustrated" – whatever words capture your feelings. Tap at the speed of three to four taps per second. Focus on your feelings while sincerely accepting yourself.

Complete the tapping sequence, take a deep breath, and ask yourself, on a scale of 1 to 10, whether the brain hunger has diminished. If the brain hunger is still at a level above 3, then go back and repeat the process, updating the phrase to reflect your current feeling about the compulsion. For example, if it has moved from overwhelming to moderate, modify the phrase as follows:

"Even though I'm experiencing moderate brain hunger, I deeply and completely accept myself."

Repeat the tapping process until the brain hunger has dropped to below three.

EFT by itself doesn't restore neural nets, but it is helpful in jolting us out of obsessive food-fantasies. Think of a car whose hydraulic brakes have failed. The car is at the top of one of those famous and very steep San Francisco hills, and without brakes, gravity will inevitably pull it down. The car will not only be out of control, but it will also create pandemonium on its way down. EFT does not restore the Naturally Thin Woman neural nets, but staying within our metaphor, it turns the car away from the hill so we have a higher likelihood of preventing damage.

Anchors Using Neuro-Linguistic Programing

An anchor is a mental coupling between a stimulus and a response; when the stimulus occurs, the response is recalled automatically by the subconscious mind. Unbeknownst to us we hold multiple anchors in our brains. For example, if we experience specific emotions listening to a certain song, those emotions will automatically come back when we listen to that song again. The advertising industry uses anchors frequently by creating a stimulus in a food commercial that triggers (in most of us) a situational hunger response.

We can develop our own anchor by coupling a chosen stimulus to a specific feeling on a consistent basis. Typically an anchor is established by using a pressure point somewhere on the body that we squeeze as we are experiencing an undesired feeling. Let's say that you want to return to a state of inner peace whenever you squeeze your left middle finger. You establish the anchor by squeezing the left middle finger every time you experience inner peace until it becomes an anchor. Once the anchor has been firmly established and you find yourself back in the tornado of compulsion, you can return to its calm eye by squeezing your left middle finger.

A possible scenario unfolds as follows. You are having a highly stressful day at work. There is no evidence of physical hunger, but you are currently wired to eat whenever you are under stress. Your stress response is to experience overwhelming emotional hunger that leads you straight to the vending machine. At this point you squeeze your left middle finger, and it allows you to experience a sense of inner peace. Inner peace and overeating are mutually exclusive, so by returning to serenity and balance you can address whatever is asking for attention.

Anchoring can be an effective tool to arrest unconscious and automatic overeating responses to the many triggers currently driving our overeating behaviors.

Chapter 6 Summary

When we are wired to overeat we must develop the equanimity to question every instance of hunger. Step 1 of the Thin Cognitive Behavior protocol is to recognize brain hunger. When we acknowledge that the hunger is non-physical, Step 2 of the protocol is to observe the symptoms of the addiction. Without disrupting the pattern, the obsessive aspect of brain hunger keeps getting stronger and stronger and is then manifested as physiological symptoms. We've compared the ability to interrupt an obsessive pattern to a mechanism responsible for shifting gears.

By interrupting the pattern, we arrest the growth of the intensity of the food thought and begin shifting brain hunger away from obsession.

Two techniques that some might find accessible and effective to interrupt the food obsession are Eye Movement Desensitization and Reprocessing (EMDR) and Emotional Freedom Technique (EFT). Both techniques have been proven effective in halting obsessive craving before it turns into compulsive eating.

Another technique is Neuro-Linguistic Programing (NLP). Using this technique we can develop an anchor to help us exit the obsessive food thought. Even the stoutest ships can drift away during a powerful storm if they're not properly anchored. An NLP anchor, such as squeezing a finger, can keep us from drifting into old, unconscious behaviors.

The reason these techniques are effective is that they help to interrupt the food obsession until we can build up our mindfulness muscles. Rewiring occurs when we are able to observe the salivation, the awakened taste buds, all of our physical responses, without being overwhelmed by them.

This page has been left intentionally blank.

Chapter 7 – What is Asking for Attention?

Tools for Step 3, Part 1: Name the Real Need

Many of us have existing programing that dominates our current eating choices and behaviors. Examples of these programs are:

a) We can't stop eating until the plate in front of us is clean.
b) In social situations, we feel compelled to eat everything offered to us. We feel it is important to please whoever is serving us, as it makes us feel emotionally connected to them.
c) We have an automatic hunger response when we begin watching a movie or sporting event.
d) Whenever we experience any emotional imbalance – be it situational, social or emotional – we are wired to find comfort in food. For some of us, the issue is deeply rooted, and only food allows us to function in an acceptable manner.

Step 3 entails two parts; Part 1 involves recognizing our current reactions, our current neural wiring that compels us to eat despite a lack of physical hunger. This recognition is essential to shift from a conditioned response. We must identify what is fueling the *situational* or *emotional* hunger, what the real need is behind it. With effort and focused mindfulness, we are going to do what the caudate nucleus should be doing easily and automatically.

Recognizing the urge to eat as situational can be as simple as looking for the usual suspects. Let me give some personal examples:

a) In the past when I worked too many hours I became hungry, as food was the only thing that made me stop working. Now I recognize that when I become hungry after working that many hours, it means that my body needs a break, and it no longer involves snacking.
b) In the past when I faced an impending deadline that was likely to be missed, I became *inexplicably* ravenous. I can now remedy what is causing the anxiety by delaying the deadline, cancelling all non-priority appointments, or notifying the affected parties that the deadline will be missed.
c) I used to eat through my anger. Today if I'm angry, I will name the source of my anger and contact friends that might hear me out or help me formulate a solution.
d) If I feel used because a friend is demanding something that will cost me time that I don't have, I can name my frustration and say, "I am so sorry, I am not able to help you at this time."
e) If I want to eat while watching a TV show, I now recognize that the show is not holding my attention, and I can turn it off.
f) If I find myself at a party where eating is the most interesting activity, I need to admit that *I'm* either not being engaging others or that I'd rather be doing something else that I find more enjoyable.
g) If I have a tough day and need to release stress, something soothing and nurturing would be helpful. Paradoxically, in this instance, food is neither

soothing nor nurturing, and if I indulge my addiction, I actually feel ashamed after overeating.

h) If anything is pushing my buttons and I feel disempowered, it's time to journal and find what is causing the discomfort.

i) If I'm devastated because I am allowing my mother/boss/husband to treat me in a non-supportive manner, I need to express my disappointment.

j) If I'm afraid that showing my feelings will be damaging to a relationship, I need to face my fears and express myself kindly but effectively.

There are many factors necessary for us to be able to name what is fueling situational hunger. Self-knowledge is paramount, as is the acceptance of our humanity – recognizing that we have emotional needs. When we are not in touch with our needs, we lack the ability to express them, let alone honor them. Even the ability to say, "*I don't know what I need, all I know is that I want to overeat, all I know is that I'm emotionally hungry*" is huge progress. Many of us lack these abilities and use food to mask the discomfort we feel when we can't meet our needs.

Let's look at some examples of social hunger:

You walk into your office to find a tray full of donuts brought in by your boss, and he is insisting that everyone must enjoy one of these treats. Your current wiring tells you that refusing the donuts would offend him … besides, they look mighty enticing. Or you could find yourself at a party with a sumptuous spread. There is recent research that indicates that when we eat with more than six people we tend to consume, on average, nearly twice as many calories as when we eat by ourselves. We are social beings, and eating is a highly social activity.

These types of situational hunger are normal responses to our desire to connect to others, and for most women, food is a vehicle to establish that connection. Once we recognize that the "hunger" is motivated by our desire for connection, we can shift our focus to an activity that fosters connection. I noticed how Naturally Thin Women inquire about recipes and express appreciation without eating. I watched many of them take one tiny bite of that tempting donut, making a fuss over how delicious it was while putting the rest away for a later treat. They related to the boss by making him feel appreciated without indulging in a donut (or three).

Prior to implementing my TCB protocol, when I lived food-obsessed, I personally witnessed a similar situation while walking in Buenos Aires with one of my naturally thin friends, Sandy. We were on our way to meet friends at an upscale restaurant for what promised to be a magnificent luncheon when we stumbled upon a most enticing bakery where chocolate croissants had just come out of the oven. What could be more tempting than the aroma of warm baked-goods? I immediately proceeded to wolf down two of those delectable treats. Sandy, who is also flesh and blood, had a different set of options available to her. After inquiring about the schedule for chocolate croissants, she consciously chose to arrive hungry at our luncheon and made plans to return to the bakery at a later date.

I was floored. How could she resist such a temptation? Was she not human? I now understand that what she experienced was not a *denial* of pleasure but a *postponement*. She was already looking forward to enjoying a great lunch with friends, and yes, while the fresh croissants were quite a temptation, indulging that urge would take away her appetite for the luncheon. She *chose* to schedule the pleasure of the warm croissant for a later time!

In contrast, once I smelled those croissants, my obsessive-compulsive mechanism was engaged. I was locked in and could not fathom any option other than the pleasure of those croissants. I experienced an overpowering craving; the reverie of gooeyness and sweetness, the fantasy that erupted in my mind was utterly mesmerizing. My choices were eating a croissant or experiencing emotionally shattering deprivation.

It is important to restate that in these social situations Naturally Thin Women do not deprive themselves; their internal mechanism allows them to name the desire to *connect* with others and to *feed* that desire without experiencing any emotional struggle. They do not forgo the food gratification, but merely postpone it to a time when they will be physically hungry. They are able to do so because it is not an either/or choice; it is not "you have it right here, right now, or forever forfeit this pleasure." It is "I *choose* to experience this pleasure at a time when I can truly be present to it."

Another form of situational hunger is triggered by our thoughts: for example, we end a challenging work day, our emotional resources have been exhausted, and we just want to be soothed. Our current wiring is that feeling soothed is tightly coupled with comfort food. Because we are eating to fill a specific need, we typically crave a specific food. We are attempting to fulfill the need to recharge with a surrogate. Food is not an effective way to satisfy anything but physical hunger. Leveraging Step 3, we would recognize our need to relax, and engage in activities that would soothe and recharge our spirits. What we find soothing is as personal and as varied as our individual preferences. For me it is walking on the beach, taking a warm bath, watching a celebration-of-life film, or experiencing soulful live music.

The last category that causes overeating is *emotional hunger*, and this category has quite a range of triggers. Once again, Step 3 begins with our willingness to name the emotional need and then determine what actions would be meaningful in addressing it. We can begin with self-dialogues such as the ones that follow.

"I am not physically hungry; I recognize that I typically take a pseudo-break by walking over to the vending machine and eating a snack, but that is my old wiring. I just need to take a break. I am going for a brisk 5-minute walk. I'm also going to take deep breaths, as I find them rejuvenating."

"I am not physically hungry; I am overwhelmed. There is no way that I can finish all of this work by next Friday. I don't know how to get all of this work completed without giving up my life. I don't know how to admit to my boss that we are not going to meet the deadline. I need to explore my options. I can either postpone the deadline or secure help. I now recognize that in the past I would anesthetize myself with food, which allowed me to suppress all of my human needs and work around the clock."

"I am not physically hungry; I am disappointed, I am angry. I can't believe that my tenants are such %^&#@!(*! I feel vulnerable that their passive-aggressive behavior might lead them to trash my house. In the past I stuffed myself to avoid these concerns and deflected my genuine feelings with self-admonishment. I have two choices: either I can confront my tenants, or I can understand that this is a business transaction, and home repairs are part of renting out a house."

If, when you read these examples, you recognize that emotional imbalance is one of your major overeating triggers, please refer to Appendix A, where we address root causes of emotional eating in detail.

Only by learning to *address* the emotional hunger instead of stuffing it with food can we truly rewire the brain and, in time, eradicate the overeating behavior. The goal is to *manage your responses* to the emotional hunger, not to control the underlying emotions themselves. Step 3 involves taking the necessary actions to honor what is asking for attention, what in the past has been suppressed. You will not only feel better, but the emotional hunger will also vanish.

Remember that sometimes the most difficult step is to diagnose the problem correctly. It might take a lot of courage to identify the root cause of unconscious eating if we have been suppressing an emotional issue for a long period of time. At the beginning, the only step possible might be to recognize, "I know that I'm not physically hungry, but all I can do when I get stressed out is eat. I currently don't have the tools to handle the stress in any meaningful manner." This is still a huge accomplishment and an important first step toward establishing Naturally Thin Woman behaviors.

A helpful strategy in recognizing situational or emotional hunger is to consciously acknowledge when we last experienced "fullness," as this allows our brain to challenge any hunger. Step 3 could then be as simple as acknowledging that we can comfortably wait to eat until lunch time, because we experienced a satisfying breakfast.

Reaching the level where you can recognize the absence of *physical hunger* and instead name it as *emotional hunger* is progress toward restoring healthy neural nets. It is infinitely better than eating automatically and not knowing – especially as it is not followed by self-loathing.

Early on, you may need a process to identify and name the root cause of the emotional hunger. The following checklist might help:

- Am I tired and I don't have the option to rest?
- Did someone push my buttons and I don't how to effectively communicate with that person?
- Am I overwhelmed because I don't know how I am going to meet all of these commitments?
- Am I anxious because I would prefer to be doing something else but I feel trapped at this event?
- Am I disappointed because the guy that I was supposed to date tonight never called, and I don't know how to express my disappointment?
- Am I angry and not allowing myself to express my rage?
- Do I feel disconnected from my community of friends and family?

On our website, thinwomanbrain.com, we have personalized assessments to further help you identify what you chronically misinterpret as emotional hunger.

Step 3, Part 2: Address What Needs Attention

Eradicating food addiction means retraining the brain. When a mental image of a food pops up and we focus on it, the normal course of action is to overeat – that's our conditioning. We must recognize the craving, give it a voice, and call it what it is: "The current wiring in my brain." Decide that you will address the need, what truly needs attention, not the craving, not the compulsion to overeat! No matter how strong the craving, observing – but not feeding – the impulse begins to rewire your brain. Every time you don't feed the craving, it speeds the rewiring process.

So I made up an experiment. The minute a food fantasy popped up, I rapidly substituted the mental image with a pleasurable image: me in Angkor Wat exploring the sights, me singing in Paris wearing a cool dress, me dancing with a bunch of friends. Any visualization where I could feel actual pleasure immediately shifted me out of the food obsession cycle.

It worked. Within minutes I lost the desire to overeat, and the food fantasy was gone. In short, I was able to influence my situational hunger by diverting my thoughts toward a pleasurable image. There was no willpower involved, just the initial intention. I worked *with* the natural processes of my brain, not *against* them.

Overeating is a learned behavior, not natural or life enhancing. Our strategy is to cause the current overeating circuitry to atrophy, which then stops the automatic response to stress, anxiety, boredom, loneliness and so forth. When the urge to fantasize about food strikes, initiate the program that will identify what is asking for attention. For those of us that have difficulty identifying our emotions, a personal checklist – similar to a pre-flight one – might be very helpful.

In order to feed what is asking for attention we must first identify that need. For many of us this might feel like a brand new skill because we have lost sensitivity to our emotional needs. It is even more difficult to identify what is asking for attention while being engulfed by an overwhelming craving. We need to find an answer to at least one of these questions:

- Is there any emotion, person, or task that I am avoiding, delaying, or dreading?
- Am I indulging in black-or-white thinking and not considering all of the possible options?
- Am I blowing the potential consequences of my current challenges out of proportion?
- Which of my needs should I attend to and nurture?

A psychologist expressed that most of the people who seek her professional help are so unaware of their feelings that they don't understand that they are eating to suppress them. When we have not developed healthy, nurturing means to deal with our feelings, eating is an automatic, unconscious response. Let's examine a handful of emotions that are typically stuffed with food.

Eating when we are bored

For many of us nighttime is when we finally have time to ourselves, *and* it's when we are most susceptible to overeating! Why is that? For most Americans, nighttime means watching television, which is laden with commercials designed to make us hungry. Furthermore, we seldom plan activities that are nurturing and truly relaxing.

Tell me, what do you have planned for tonight that is life-enhancing, contributes to your goals, and is aligned with your dreams?

Our relationship with food is our relationship with our inner self. Food substitutes for loving connections, engaging activities, spiritual meaning, even our search for purpose. Part of the process that eradicates food addiction is changing the responses that our brain generates when thinking about food. It is the ability to acknowledge when our activity is not engaging instead of calling it boredom!

One of my all-time favorite quotes is:

Only boring people get bored.

And once we acknowledge we are *bored*, we have to muster the courage to recognize that boredom is a form of self-rejection. Food is how we attempt to satisfy emotional needs when we are not living a life that we find fulfilling. Eating when we are *bored* is nothing but an excuse to stuff down our soul's calling. If we were listening to our innermost needs we would never be bored. Yes, we could say:

- I don't feel engaged or connected to anyone at this party.
- I am not finding this movie/TV show/play entertaining.
- Instead of this activity, I would rather be home working on my project.

Once we muster the courage to be completely honest and recognize that we are not engaged, then it's time to exit the party, turn off the tube, leave the activity, and pursue those projects that really feed our soul. When we are enthusiastically pursuing our heart's deepest desires we don't experience boredom.

Eating when we are lonely

Loneliness is rooted in the belief that we are not worth loving: "I am flawed. No one could ever love me." It is not about being alone, it is about feeling undesirable. Recognizing the difference between feeling unlovable and feeling deserted, like no one is there for you, is important.

Feeling unlovable is a matter of self-worth. Yes, there are times when we long to share our sorrows, successes, concerns, or just process our day with another – someone close to us – and they are not available. But it is important to recognize the difference between our inability to reach someone when we need them and our being intrinsically unlovable; it helps us to recognize why we feel a void. Instead of stuffing this void with food we can express our need for connection via an email, journaling, or even a long voicemail.

If, however, the issue is chronic, perhaps it's time to investigate why people are not there for us. But know this: loneliness is not cured with food. In fact, when we do resort to food, the end result is shame. Food may be warm, but it doesn't provide warmth; it may be comforting but it doesn't soothe. When we eat because we tell ourselves we are lonely, we end up feeling ashamed.

Eating because of the blues

Feeling blue is that emotional state when we have lost perspective about our options. Most of us have a myriad of options, but when we experience the blues, we fall into a lethargic stupor and sit around hoping that something will spark our interest. Contrary to popular belief, action precedes motivation. Instead of waiting until we feel motivated, we need to get up and do something. To start, do anything first!

It could be a small act of kindness or doing something nice for yourself: relaxing in a bath, lighting an aromatherapy candle, compiling a playlist, or giving yourself a pedicure. Alternatively, you could do some small task around the house: laundry, organizing a drawer, emptying the dishwasher – anything that feels easily doable and leads you to experience a sense of achievement.

But know this, when we eat because we have the blues, it's not going to make us feel better. It's just the opposite. At the end of the overeating cycle we always feel bad, we feel ashamed. Remember that the addiction is not just to the food but to the cycle of shame.

Eating because we are tired

Feeling tired typically has two sources: our activity level is too low or the quality of our sleep is poor. Paradoxically, the less activity we have, the more lethargic we feel, and we are constantly tired. Most people continue to believe that they should exercise to lose weight. In fact, it takes a tremendous amount of effort to lose weight via exercise. However exercise does restore a higher sense of well-being; otherwise we are chronically tired.

The second cause for chronic tiredness is poor sleeping patterns. This is typically caused by a mind that has difficulty becoming quiet, possibly rooted in chronic stress. Elevated levels of stress then lead to poor sleep patterns, which perpetuates the cycle of feeling tired. Chronic stress is the body's fight-or-flight response, and it generates a large amount of cortisol. Cortisol makes you retain fat! This becomes a vicious cycle: lack of sleep → tiredness → stress →cortisol → overeating → tiredness → poor sleep. You get the picture, it's never-ending.

Furthermore, there are now scores of studies that identify that chronic sleep deprivation increases the likelihood of overeating and interferes with how the body and the brain use our main source of energy, glucose. Sleep deprivation leaves us feeling drained and understandably craving sweets or anything else that has a chance to restore our energy level.

A single night with little sleep lowers the amount of blood to the prefrontal cortex; in fact sleep researchers call it a "mild prefrontal dysfunction." The body actually gets stuck in a physiological fight-or-flight state, and there are measurably higher levels of stress hormones, which then increase our stress level.

The comprehensive solution is to address the root cause of the stress. We must challenge any beliefs that lead to a stressful life: I'm Superwoman, my plate is always full, I don't have time to exercise or meditate or eat healthily, I have an obligation to maintain relationships that I don't find nurturing. Once again, and perhaps this is beating a dead horse, meditation is one of the best investments we can make to manage stress. Meditation affords us equanimity, clarity and perspective. A stressful lifestyle causes sleep deprivation, which then leads to overeating.

Eating when we are disappointed

Sadness and surprise are the key components of disappointment. It seems to arise out of our own expectations or demands about how we think the world should be or how we think people should act. In other words, disappointment is a misaligned view of reality. Looking at it this way could help us accept that we didn't really understand things as well as we thought or that perhaps our expectations were unrealistic. It is easier for us to take responsibility and thus to reduce its intensity when view from this perspective. It also helps us avoid laying guilt trips. Instead of using the word "disappointed," we might substitute the word "dissatisfied," which reminds us that what we are responding to is our own *interpretation* of the external events.

A more intense form of disappointment is bitterness, which tells us that not only did we expect something, but we blame someone else for the fact that we didn't get it. For some of us, this happens fairly frequently. We got passed over for a raise or promotion. Our pregnancy test came out negative again. Our fiancé didn't show up for the wedding.

Of course, these examples represent situations that will result in different degrees of disappointment and lead to a wide range of emotions. But the basic experience of disappointment is the same. For most people, two questions arise: first, how do I avoid being disappointed? Second, what do I do when I experience disappointment?

Our society focuses on avoiding disappointment, and most overeaters use food as their key avoidance strategy. The issue is compounded if you are a control freak. When you don't have control over everything in the world; the result is disappointment. Your *expectations*, however, are within your ability to control, or at least to manage.

Psychologists also recommend learning to self-soothe. But many of us don't do it well, or in all circumstances. Self-soothing, at a very basic level, is providing yourself with a feeling of physical comfort. You see this with children in actions like thumb-sucking, rocking, or holding a blanket or stuffed animal. For an adult, a healthy expression of disappointment is to give it full voice without shame or guilt.

Communicating disappointment in a non-blaming way is a very useful skill to develop. You communicate with the person who you believe is the source of the disappointment so that you can learn their perspective. For example, you would probably feel less disappointed that a friend missed your lunch date if you discovered that she had a personal issue come up as she was leaving her house. If you just get angry and refuse to return her phone calls, you will never know what happened.

Addressing our Emotional Needs

What action can potentially address the real need? Here are a few suggestions.

Feeling	Possible Action Plan
The blues	Remind yourself that you've lost perspective; any task that returns you to a state of gratitude will evaporate the blues. Do something nice for yourself. NOW. Complete a small project.
Boredom	Remember that boredom is a form of self-rejection. It is important to work on one of your dream projects, work on a vision board, reconnect and re-invest in your life's calling. If you don't know what your life's calling is, make a commitment to discover it. There are thousands of resources and workbooks to assist you on that quest, so shift your energies toward that discovery process.
Disappointment	Do a reality check with anyone involved. Call a friend, journal, or scream!
Tiredness	If you overeat due to chronic sleep deprivation, invest in a meditation practice, because it quiets the monkey mind. One hour prior to going to sleep start your "shut down" cycle, with relaxing music, a soothing bath, sensual pajamas, low lights, no computer time, reading (as long as it's not a thriller or adventure) – in short, forfeit anything that increases your excitement level.
Loneliness	Call a friend. Do something nice for someone, even if it is a stranger. Go to a hospice or child crisis center and lend a hand.
Anger	If it's chronic anger, get therapy from a professional with expertise in anger management. If it's occasional anger, give it loud voice, punch a bag while you express your anger, or go for a run.
Stress	Run or do some vigorous exercise. Look at the bigger picture and gain perspective. Meditate. ☺ You have two choices: to indulge in worst-case scenario thinking (and increase your stress) or entertain options that go beyond black-or-white.

If you are having a difficult time identifying your feeling, do a breathing exercise, (refer to Conscious Breathing in Chapter 5) and reconnect with your body. Keep inquiring gently, "What is asking for attention? What am I feeling? How is my energy level?"

What's important is to make a change, using physical exercise or meditation, playing music you like, or recording your feelings in a journal. It doesn't matter, as long as it's something that you can do immediately, instead of unconsciously overeating – the goal is to experience a shift toward the true need. Be prepared to repeat the activity as often as necessary. If, for some reason, you are constrained and can't execute the alternative activity, *imagine* yourself doing it, step by step, with hearty intention.

It is vital to challenge the belief that emotional needs can be satisfied with food, that eating is going to make you feel better. Think about it: you are lonely and overeating is going to provide companionship? You are disappointed and eating is going to rectify the situation? You are bored and eating is going to entertain you? Keep reminding yourself that the one sure feeling overeating *will* cause is shame. Anytime we overeat what we feel is ashamed, so at its core, food addiction returns us to the cycle of shame. (We'll talk more about the cycle of shame in Appendix A.)

Chapter 7 Summary

Step 3 has two parts: Part 1 is the ability to *Name the Need* that is manifesting itself as brain hunger. Non-physical hunger has many triggers, including social situations and emotional imbalances. Social triggers lead us to believe that we must eat to fit in or where we are uncomfortable and believe that we will feel better by eating. Emotional hunger is triggered when we can't name or don't know how to address our emotional needs, or we have not yet developed the ability to self-soothe.

As our mindfulness increases and we develop an understanding of our needs, the length between episodes of brain hunger will grow longer, until one day it will be history.

Part 2 of Step 3 is the ability to address whatever need is masquerading as hunger. Sometimes this is not a trivial step, and all we can verbalize is: "*I don't know how to address my emotional need, and in the past I have used food.*" The good news is that once we are able to identify what is asking for attention, we can develop the skills to address the true need instead of suppressing it. When we overeat, we continue to feed the cycle of shame. In having the courage to name the underlying need and address it, we are actually strengthening our healthy neural nets.

Chapter 8 – Restoring Food as Nourishment

Forbidden Foods

One of the major fallacies in weight-loss strategies is avoiding or minimizing entire categories of foods (fat, carbs, sugar, etc.). What we finally understand is that categorizing foods as *forbidden* plunges the brain into further food obsession. It is counterproductive to establishing healthy eating behaviors. The reason is simple: as long as we believe that these foods are "forbidden," they will retain a high emotional charge, similar to the power of an illicit love affair. Marking these foods as forbidden creates the polar bear effect (as we discussed in Chapter 2) and is actually detrimental, as it causes us to constantly fantasize about them. There's something in human nature that wants what it can't have. Researchers call this the *forbidden fruit hypothesis*. The moment that we experience ego depletion, the moment we have a challenging day where we need to be soothed or comforted, like a moth to a light, we uncontrollably binge on these "forbidden foods." That explains the frenzy and voracity with which we eat these foods once our suppression mechanism is exhausted.

Cognitive research has shown that exposure to food triggers, paired with coaching in response-prevention, is an extremely effective technique for rewiring the brain. After we learn how to eat in a non-compulsive manner, we can then introduce "forbidden foods." Once we trust that we can eat mindfully, it is of the utmost importance that we eat *whatever the hell we want.* When we do, a miracle happens! We choose to eat nurturing and energizing foods, even "forbidden foods," but we do so without *over*eating.

The solution is to use the TCB protocol to master eating mindfully, even if at first it is mechanical. I'll share my experience. During my days of mindless eating, I would not allow myself to have nachos or ice cream in the house. But lo and behold, after a particularly challenging day at the office, I typically stopped at the grocery store and – you guessed it – bought a couple of bags of nacho chips and a tub of ice cream. I would then overindulge in these forbidden foods. The moment the binge concluded I would beat myself up. The next day I would give the remaining ice cream and nacho chips to a friend. This is a scene that repeated itself countless times.

After I understood the implication of *ego depletion* (defined in Chapter 2), combined with the *forbidden fruit hypothesis,* my history of suppression and bingeing finally made sense. I then made it a point to plan several meals where nachos were the main event; I made nachos supreme, ordered nacho platters at restaurants, and invented my own recipes for nachos laden with healthful toppings. After a week of nacho festivities, the bags of tortilla chips could sit around the kitchen without causing me any anxiety or struggle. I now have to throw them away because they go stale; they no longer hold any mystical power over me.

Talk to Naturally Thin Women and you will find that they always say, "I eat whatever I want." The basic skill is to eat in a mindful manner, without forbidding any food. In fact, I no longer have *any* forbidden food categories.

On our website, our personalized programs include specific protocols for rewiring the brain around the topic of forbidden foods.

Healthy or Food-Obsessed Brain

The human species has populated planet Earth for just one million years. During these thousand millennia we initially sustained ourselves as meat-eaters, slowly evolving into agrarian societies. However, these types of eating changes were evolutionary; they occurred over thousands of years.

The earliest reference we find in literature about dieting dates back to the 1820s. However, it was not until the 1960s that the concept of *diet foods* was widely introduced. The low-carb diet was invented in 1972 by cardiologist Robert C. Atkins, M.D. This was followed in the 1990s by the low-fat diet, for which Susan Powter was the most ardent spokesperson.

In order to produce an enticing low-fat version of naturally fatty items, the food industry added substantial amounts of sugar. If you compare most *low-fat* foods with their *natural* counterparts, you'll find that the sugar content is astronomical. To solve the problem that was instigated by the low-fat food industry we have recently moved to a *low-sugar* diet, as espoused by Jorge Cruise.

With the advent of diet foods we have embraced the black-or-white thinking that demonizes certain categories of foods. We have gone through phases of low-carb, fat-free, and low-sugar diets, and we are now back to counting calories. Think about it: of the 50,000 generations of humans, only the last three have bought into the concept of diet foods. The paradox is that we are fueling a $63 billion/year diet industry in the United States, the country with the fattest population on the planet. What is it that they say about insanity?

In parallel with the diet-food explosion, we have elevated convenience (how much time it takes to prepare food) to a critical, necessary consideration. For the sake of saving time, we are now offered a wide selection of packaged, frozen, and canned foods. Only 15% of most supermarket aisles are dedicated to fresh food, much of which is inundated with chemicals.

Everyone has heard the phrase "you are what you eat." However, few of us understand the connection between *eating* healthy and *staying* thin. Advertising and supermarket displays lure us into choosing low-cost over healthy alternatives. The irony is that we limit our grocery budget while paying extravagant amounts for pharmaceuticals to keep us "healthy." Most consumers are ignorant of what truly nourishes their bodies. And it is not "one size fits all." Each Naturally Thin Woman recognizes what foods make her feel alive and vibrant and what foods make her feel sluggish and weighed down.

But here is the bottom line: eating over-processed foods contributes to food obsession! Any flavor-enhanced food is meant to heighten the pleasure experience. As discussed in the section entitled *Wired to Overeat*, "enhanced" foods have compromised the brain mechanism that generates a healthy level of dopamine. Our ability to re-experience pleasure when eating *natural* foods might require a detox period. It might be necessary to recalibrate our palates away from the highly processed flavors that we currently crave. Think about it: if the idea of eating the very foods that ensure your thinness doesn't sound appealing, what caused that aversion? Why is it that we can't experience pleasure when eating healthful foods? How did we learn that life-enhancing foods were not appetizing?

Part of our journey back to wholesome eating includes relearning to enjoy the foods that restore our Naturally Thin Woman neural nets. Our ability to stay the course is based on the power of our self-advocacy. When we start craving healthful foods, the excuses of "I don't have time to prepare a nutritious meal" or "I don't see the value of investing in 'health foods'" must be faced squarely and replaced by a nurturing and loud response: "I love to feel good!" I DESERVE IT!

Here is a fantastic question:

If money were not an issue and you had a full-time cook, what eating plan would you choose? Would your menu include meals that are tasty, made with foods that:

a) Help you shed pounds easily?
b) Promote overall health?
c) Increase your energy level?

What would you be willing to invest to get back to optimum health, where you feel energized all the time?

Releasing the Extra Weight

If you are carrying extra pounds, the assessment tools on our website incorporate the latest scientific findings regarding weight loss, including the benefits of weight training. On our website we also offer support programs that strive to address your specific level of addiction while accounting for your challenges and lifestyle.

Nutrients that Promote Neuroplasticity

Substances such as glutathione, selenium, fish oil and B-complex have been documented as helpful in the construction of neural nets. We discuss these nutrients within the personalized assessments on our website.

Healing the Famine Brain

My forbidden foods used to be nachos, pizza, subs, and ice cream. By forbidding them, I had wired myself to believe that I could never have them again, which effectively plunged the brain into deeper food obsession. Once I reached ego depletion, or whenever I would get stressed out, these were the exact foods I had to grab and eat compulsively, as fast and as much as I could. That explains the frenzy, eating directly out of the refrigerator, or eating in the car the moment that I got them.

Reintroducing these forbidden foods was an exorcising process, one where the foods were disarmed so that my brain could heal. I had to learn how to eat these foods in a state of centeredness, deliberately, where my brain could accept that it was OK to have them. The message I had to assimilate was: "You can eat these foods as frequently as you would like. They will always be here. There is nothing special about these foods. You can enjoy them whenever you like."

As you read this, you might feel panicked or intrigued: how is it possible to eat foods typically associated with gaining weight? Keeping forbidden foods in the house goes against the advice of 99% of the diet gurus, as they believe that it is the food that triggers the binge cycle. This advice, while well intentioned, is counter to healing famine brain. Healing famine brain is an essential aspect in restoring the Naturally Thin Woman neural nets.

Increasing Dopamine Level

In search of the dopamine fix, we keep eating and eating in the hope of getting our high. However, as discussed in Chapter 3, once our dopamine mechanism is faulty we tend to eat larger and larger amounts of foods before we are able to experience pleasure. The following recommendations have been shown to improve dopamine production. Again, some individuals experience zero dopamine improvement, as their genes inhibit the breakdown of certain amino acids.

1 – Eat foods rich in tyrosine. Almonds, avocados, bananas, low-fat dairy, lima beans, sesame seeds and pumpkin seeds may all help the body to produce more dopamine.

2 – Increase your intake of antioxidants. Dopamine oxidizes easily, and antioxidants may reduce free radical damage in the brain cells that produce dopamine. Many fruits and vegetables are rich in antioxidants:

- Beta-carotene and carotenoids: Orange vegetables and fruits, leafy greens, asparagus, broccoli
- Vitamin C: Peppers, papaya, citrus fruits, strawberries, cauliflower, Brussels sprouts, broccoli
- Vitamin E: Almonds, sunflower seeds, wheat germ oil, greens

3 – Avoid food that interferes with healthy brain function. Such foods typically are highly processed and include added sugar, flavor enhancers, hydrogenated oils, caffeine, and saturated fats.

Please note that flavor-enhanced foods are likely to cause overeating. It is highly, highly recommended to consume non-processed versions of whatever food it is that you want to eat. Just think about it, the flavors were added to stimulate the pleasure centers of the brain. But in the process of enjoying the taste of the additives, we compromise our ability to discern when we are satiated. A child is not likely to tell you that she has had enough candy.

4 – Invest in aerobic exercise to keep dopamine levels healthy. Aerobics increases blood calcium, which stimulates dopamine production and uptake in your brain. Try 30 to 60 minutes of power walking, dancing, vigorous swimming, or jogging to jump-start your dopamine.

5 – Get plenty of sleep. Your brain uses very little dopamine while you sleep, which helps you to build up your supply naturally for the next day. Eight hours of sleep per night continues to be recommended.

6 – Meditate. Yet another benefit of meditation is that it can increase dopamine production by up to 65%!

7 – Supplements. Some physicians recommend Vitamin B6 supplements and L-phenylalanine to elevate dopamine in the brain. You can buy most of these at your local store.

8 – Antidepressants. Low dopamine levels are sometimes associated with depression. You can talk to your doctor about starting an antidepressant if natural methods don't work to relieve symptoms of low energy.

Chapter 8 Summary

For a Naturally Thin Woman, food is nourishment, food is pleasure, and food is restorative.

The forbidden foods that most overeaters hold in guarded secrecy are counterproductive. Once we learn to eat mindfully, we can enjoy these forbidden foods without fear of over-indulging and reverting back to old habits. Our relationship to those foods will have changed, and will have healed to a point where we are able to enjoy them without fear.

As opposed to the latest low-this, diet-that, one-size-fits-all trends, it would be better if we could trust what our body craves and nurture those preferences mindfully. That way we can each find what genuinely nourishes our body and soul.

This page has been left intentionally blank.

Chapter 9 – Failure to Plan is Planning to Fail

Ending the Madness

After many, many months of working inhumane hours and giving up everything in my personal life at another corporate gig, I finally had the courage to weigh myself. For the 11th time in my life I stared at a number on the scale that I could hardly believe. My closet was once more full of size 18 to 22 clothes. How could this have happened again? I felt like I was caught in Dante's Inferno, in an endless loop, a labyrinth where, after walking for miles, I found myself exactly where I had started. This was so familiar, and once again I was determined to fight myself back to a single-digit size.

However, this time was different. What finally dawned on me was a simple question: Why should I pursue any weight loss program without understanding why I always gain all of the weight back? So I paused and acknowledged that without first healing the food obsession, the compulsion with which I ate, I was just buying into another con, signing up for another failure. What is it that the Irish say? "Fool me once shame on you, fool me twice…" I knew that whenever I undertook a new diet approach I would lose weight; I knew it to the core of my being, because that had been my experience so many previous times. But finally I formulated the Satori question: When this weight comes off (again), what makes me believe that it will stay off? What am I doing differently from what I have done the previous 11 times?

At that point in my awareness I didn't have an answer, but I committed not to blindly buy into the latest "Eat Less, Move More" weight-loss philosophy until I understood what was different about Naturally Thin Women. This chapter will cover what has been proven scientifically as the most effective, healthy, and meaningful way to lose weight. In case there is any doubt, we must state once again that the practice of eating only certain foods and engaging in an exercise program should not be pursued until your Naturally Thin Woman's neural nets are restored.

Phases of Rewiring

The measure of success, what indicates that you have restored your Naturally Thin Woman's brain, can be summarized in one characteristic, mindful eating: You eat only when you are physically hungry and you can enjoy the experience for what it is, nourishment and pleasure. You eat whatever the hell you want. You eat slowly and calmly, putting the fork down between bites, chewing until it is mush in your mouth, taking at least one breath in between bites. You don't miss the piranha-like frenzy when you used to shovel food as fast as you could into your mouth. You can truly enjoy the experience, you can tell when your taste buds lose pleasure, and you trust that this is your body telling you that it has had enough. You know that you can eat in another 3 to 4 hours, so eating small portions does not create any anxiety. When you completely and unambiguously trust your body's messages, when you are able to experience genuine satisfaction eating small portions, you have not only mastered mindful eating, you've restored your healthy brain.

Mastering mindful eating, like the acquisition of any new skill, has two components. First is the mechanical practice to gain the skill and second is the emotional aspect of changing our feelings about the food. As we practice this new skill, we experience evidence of progress, and then one day, Kazam! Food no longer has any power over us. Like learning how to play the piano, or how to French-braid hair, the beginning feels awkward and contrived. Let's discuss the five phases of reclaiming our birthright and restoring our Naturally Thin Woman's brain.

Within each of the five phases there are six areas where we will experience a tangible change, an awareness or progress. These are:

1. **Our brain wiring** – Our involuntary reaction to food is driven by our existing neural wiring. Within our brain there is a measureable activity when we fantasize about food, when we experience external triggers, or after consuming highly addictive foods, etc. If we could take before-and-after fMRIs at the beginning of the rewiring and after our Naturally Thin neural nets have been restored, there would be a significant difference in brain activity and amount of dopamine.

2. **Our self-knowledge** – We gain higher and higher awareness of the involuntary, hardwired behaviors. We recognize these physical reactions as tangible manifestations of the addiction. As we know from the TCB protocol, when we can observe some of these involuntary, hardwired behaviors without compulsion or anxiety, that is a sign that rewiring is occurring.

3. **Our recognition of physical hunger** – As the Naturally Thin Woman neural nets restore, we will more easily discern the difference between physical and brain hunger.

4. **Our awareness of emotional imbalance** – Since for many women emotional imbalance is *the* prominent trigger to overeating, being able to recognize when we are out of balance is critical.

5. **Our mindfulness practice** – Mindfulness is what allows us to rewire, and the goal is to experience progress in this area.

6. **Our awareness of the cycle of shame** – Many of us are unaware that we overeat not just to feel pleasure but to also experience the negative feelings that come after overeating. We are wired to preserve the belief that we are fundamentally flawed. Gaining a deeper understanding of the cycle of shame is tremendously helpful in restoring the Naturally Thin Woman wiring.

Each phase measures progress in either modeling a specific behavior or achieving a higher level of awareness. These are the indicators that we are moving to the next phase.

Phase of Wiring	Objectives
1 – Clueless **Wiring** – Our brain is food-obsessed, we are wired to overeat, yet we have zero awareness as to the mechanisms that drive our overeating and its root causes. Unforeseen situations and challenging emotions trigger unexpected hunger. **Self-Knowledge** – We are not even aware that we think about food so frequently. We are clueless that there are many triggers that cause us to overeat. We are oblivious that being food-obsessed is not natural. **Non-Physical Hunger** – We are unaware that there is such a thing as brain hunger, let alone its subtle variations and triggers. We experience hunger simply as an overwhelming drive that rules our lives. TV commercials, food at the office, feeling out of our comfort zone in a social setting – all of these trigger a compulsion to overeat. **Emotional Imbalance** – Whenever we experience an emotional challenge, we lack the self-knowledge and the basic ability to address our emotional needs. The lack of awareness is significant, in some cases reflecting deeply rooted emotional issues. Overeating is what initiates the cycle of shame, which keeps us from making progress in our emotional development. **Mindfulness Practice** – We have zero awareness that our brains are overheating because of our obsessive food thoughts. We are not aware that there is a correlation between a mindfulness practice and our ability to stop fueling the food obsession. In many cases the mere idea of practices such as meditation causes a high level of anxiety. **Cycle of Shame** – We possess zero awareness that the root of our addiction is a return to the cycle of shame. At a	**Become Aware** ✓ We become aware as to how we became: food-obsessed and powerless around certain foods. ✓ We observe as our brains switch from daily events to obsessing about food. ✓ We understand why forbidden foods trigger a binge. ✓ We understand that once our stress reaches a high level, the equanimity necessary to merely observe certain foods without salivating is obliterated. Our brain automatically overheats, and eating becomes a physical mandate. ✓ We accept that while our brain is food-obsessed we are as likely to avoid overeating as we are likely to hold our breath for 10 minutes. These are skills that can be acquired, but only after some training. Currently our brain is wired to overeat, and once it is rattled, every single mechanism that drives our biological imperative will be engaged to make us overeat. ✓ At this phase our goal is not to lose weight. Instead, we strive to become conscious and accept that "eat less, move more" should be attempted only after we have mastered equanimity and self-advocacy. There are five phases to the rewiring process; the first phase is to become aware.

The Thin Woman's Brain

Phase of Wiring	Objectives
gut level we believe that we are inadequate and unworthy, so experiencing the shame after a binge is our way of keeping those beliefs alive by reinforcing them.	

2 – Intellectual Recognition

Wiring – Our brain is food-obsessed, we are wired to overeat, but we now intellectually understand the rewiring process, the TCB protocol, and the promise of lowering our anxiety around social, emotional, or situational triggers.

Self-Knowledge – Even though we are still wired to overeat and we still obsess about food on a fairly frequent basis, we are able to recognize and accept the difference between physical hunger and other types of hunger.

Non-Physical Hunger – We are still compelled to eat even when not physically hungry. It is helpful to understand the TCB protocol, but mere intellectual awareness does not restore Naturally Thin Woman neural nets. We still become "hungry" when presented with situational opportunities or emotional triggers, for example, walking by a bakery. However we begin to accept that it is not physical hunger.

Emotional imbalance – Whenever there is an emotional imbalance we are able to recognize our human needs, perhaps even distinguish the different tone of these emotions, even though we have not yet developed the self-advocacy to address the underlying need. We have not yet strengthened the emotional muscle to self-soothe, and our current recourse is overeating.

Mindfulness practice – We intellectually understand the benefit of mindfulness practices but still experience high anxiety, and therefore a lack of success, when attempting them.

Recognition and Acceptance

✓ Despite high anxiety we begin a mindfulness practice.

✓ We begin to develop awareness as to when we become food-obsessed: What was the situation, emotional trigger, social anxiety, etc.?

✓ We increase our ability to clearly recognize brain hunger as social, situational, or emotional in nature.

✓ We accept our humanity, which entails accepting our many emotional needs, short-comings, and propensity to make mistakes.

✓ We invest in any book, workshop, or one-on-one therapy that allows us to develop self-knowledge and the emotional muscle to self-soothe.

✓ We identify any social gatherings that trigger obsessive food thoughts or that might not be contributing to our sense of well-being.

✓ We become aware of any stress triggers. What beliefs, tasks, or responsibilities, if modified, would reduce our stress level?

✓ It is critical to eat whatever we want, especially forbidden foods. Paradoxically, these forbidden foods are the ones that hold the key to arriving at equanimity. The shift is to eat them mindfully until they no longer cause anxiety and until we stop running to them whenever we experience high stress. At the beginning it is

Phase of Wiring	Objectives
Cycle of Shame – We intellectually understand the addiction to the cycle of shame, but without the ability to eat mindfully, we still feel ashamed every time we overeat.	difficult to believe, but it *is* possible to eat forbidden foods mindfully.
3 - Novice **Wiring** – We are still wired to overeat but begin to experience less anxiety and show measurable, albeit minor, improvements in our ability to eat mindfully. **Self-Knowledge** – We accept our humanity, our need to experience the entire spectrum of negative emotions. We have made a commitment to recognize our triggers and to learn what we find helpful and soothing in order to address our emotional needs. We commit to investing in the practices, books, personal therapy, or workshops that allow us to have a healthy emotional life. **Non-Physical Hunger** – We recognize the difference between physical hunger and emotional, situational, or social hunger. We accept that we might still overeat even when we are not physically hungry. However, we now recognize the compulsion to overeat as a stress reaction or an emotional imbalance caused by any challenges or discomfort in our life. We now understand the power that forbidden foods hold over us, and we begin incorporating these foods into our daily diet. There is some struggle when eating these foods, but the anxiety level is lower. **Emotional imbalance** – We begin to recognize and are able to name anger, disappointment, loneliness, boredom, fatigue, the blues, or any emotion that in the past triggered overeating. At this phase we might only be able to name those emotions (especially while our brain is still overheating) however it is	**Establish Mindfulness** ✓ We begin a mindfulness practice that allows us to restore the Naturally Thin Woman neural nets. ✓ We are able to verbally express our preferences and personal needs. ✓ We are able to identify the people and activities that bring us joy and those that we feel are a chore or that create stress. ✓ We begin to experience social, emotional or situational hunger, naming it and being able to address what is asking for attention. ✓ We are able to eat mindfully even when we experience some anxiety. ✓ We are able to experience anger, disappointment, boredom, or the blues and have the ability to accept these human needs without resorting to food. ✓ We are aware that when we overeat it will trigger the cycle of shame.

Phase of Wiring	Objectives
important to measure our progress. **Mindfulness practice** – At this phase we know that it is infinitely more meaningful to achieve equanimity than to count calories. This understanding allows us to invest in a mindfulness practice, as we thoroughly understand its benefits. We now accept that when our stress level is high we are hardwired to experience anxiety around forbidden foods. We are able to consistently invest in a mindfulness practice.	
Cycle of Shame – We recognize that any time we overeat we will experience shame. We begin examining where these beliefs of unworthiness started.	

4 - Proficiency

Wiring – We spend less and less of our day fantasizing about food. We are able to experience decreased anxiety around food, even forbidden foods.

Emotional Imbalance – We begin to name and accept the emotions that previously sent us flying non-stop to the vending machine or the refrigerator. We begin to recognize, even anticipate, all of the emotional events that previously pushed our buttons, and we are willing to seek meaningful outlets instead of overeating.

Non-Physical Hunger – We are able to tolerate longer and longer periods around sumptuous food without becoming anxious and without feeling an overpowering drive to overeat. We unequivocally recognize the difference between physical hunger and other types of hunger.

Emotional Imbalance – We accept our emotions, all of them. We have developed meaningful ways of dealing with our emotional challenges.

Mindfulness Practice – There is no resistance to our mindfulness practice as we know it as the best investment of our time. We experience longer and

Experience Progress

✓ Because we are experiencing steady progress, it is becoming easier and easier to conduct mindfulness practices for longer periods.

✓ It is becoming easier and easier to eat mindfully.

✓ It is becoming easier and easier to acknowledge and name our emotional needs and challenges.

✓ It is becoming easier and easier to differentiate between social, emotional, and situational hunger versus physical hunger.

✓ Whenever we experience an emotional imbalance or challenge we are able to address what is asking for attention without resorting to food.

✓ The belief that we are essentially flawed and inadequate grows weaker and weaker. We stop feeding the cycle of shame.

Phase of Wiring	Objectives
longer periods of equanimity which support our ability to eat mindfully and without anxiety. **Cycle of Shame** – We continue to invest time exploring our addiction to the cycle of shame and we discover how to eradicate whatever created our beliefs of unworthiness.	
5 – Naturally Thin **Wiring** – We are able to eat mindfully with no anxiety around food and zero stress about the possibility of overeating. We experience zero anxiety in the presence of a sumptuous smorgasbord; an awkward social situation does not make us feel inexplicably hungry. We can self-soothe and address emotional needs without the desire to overeat. We hate feeling bloated. **Self-Knowledge** – We fully accept our humanity and our emotional needs. **Non-Physical Hunger** – There is zero compulsion to overeat, as overeating is no longer strongly coupled with experiencing pleasure. We recognize the difference between physical hunger and emotional, social, and situational food triggers. **Emotional imbalance** – Whenever we experience the ups and downs of life, we address what is asking for attention without experiencing inexplicable hunger. **Mindfulness practice** – One of our life priorities is our mindfulness practice, which we accept as the foundation to remain in a state of equanimity. **Cycle of Shame** – We have given up using food to feel inadequate and we no longer feed the cycle of shame.	**Lifelong Thinness** ✓ Only *physical hunger* prompts us to eat. ✓ We enjoy food – without obsessing, without conflict, and without trauma. ✓ We make time to enjoy our meals. ✓ We can assess our needs against our food options. ✓ We dislike the physical discomfort of feeling bloated or stuffed. ✓ We eat whatever we want while considering the impact of calories. ✓ Food is not our primary source of joy. ✓ We are attuned to the natural rhythm of the day, and we let that guide our eating. ✓ We are able to experience the ups and downs of life without feeling hungry. ✓ We are able to lose weight by following a healthy eating regimen, without plunging our brain back into food obsession. The moment we experience food in the manner described in Phase 5, we have restored our Naturally Thin Woman neural nets.

Stress-Proofing Your Brain

In 2007 the American Psychological Association reported that 43% of Americans overeat when stressed, which begs the question, why do so many of us respond to stress by running to the refrigerator? What neuroscientists are now documenting is that those of us who have a history of dieting are 98% more likely to overeat in response to stress. Most of us are aware that chronic stress lowers our quality of life – it disrupts sleep, increases anxiety level, lowers our effectiveness and causes or exacerbates scores of physical challenges.

Many scientists attribute unhealthy levels of stress to:

- **Personal relationships** – Ineffective communication, lack of shared values
- **Over-commitment** – Ego depletion, no time allotted to recharge our batteries
- **Anxiety over finances**
- **Too much information** – We simply are not meant to be plugged in 24/7
- **Lack of silence in our lives** – No quiet space to be able to think and feel
- **Glucose plunge** – Poor management of blood-sugar level, which leads to irritability, headaches, and exhaustion
- **Traumatic scars** – Unaddressed abuse can trigger stressful reactions

Most of us have read the many magazine articles that encourage us to manage these triggers by:

1. Developing effective communication skills or minimizing interaction with non-nurturing people; in some extreme cases, ending toxic relationships.
2. Managing your over-commitments by bagging them, bartering them, or bettering them. Bagging is simple: If you don't love to do something, and you don't have to do it, don't do it. To barter a task, find someone who loves doing what you hate, and who dislikes something you like, then swap activities. Commitments that can't be bagged or bartered can usually be bettered. If you're tired of going to a shopping mall but really want to choose gifts yourself, use catalogs or the Internet.
3. Promoting any practice that contributes to your ability to manage your stress level, making it the highest priority in your daily calendar.
4. Living within your means – setting a budget, getting financial management help if necessary.
5. Investing the time for mindfulness practice – meditation, long-distance running, T'ai Chi, and ocean swimming are a few examples.
6. Having healthy food and healthy eating practices – investing the time to shop, cook, and maintain healthy blood-sugar levels. Eating mindfully.
7. Addressing trauma. There are wise friends, gifted therapists, issue-specific workshops, and online resources that are helpful. What typically is lacking is the courage to face the dragon.

Stanford neuroendocrinologist Robert Sapolsky, Ph.D., has spent over 30 years studying the effects of prolonged, sustained, and excessive stress. For 99% of our human history, stress was three minutes of screaming terror in the savannah, after which you had either outrun the danger or ended up as lunch. That is genuine stress compared to what today we manufacture in our heads. But those biological systems are still active and are overwhelming whether we create the stress ourselves or not. Dr. Sapolsky catalogued the leading triggers for this mental reaction:

- For many people the primary source of stress is work-related. The lower you are in the hierarchy, the less powerful you feel and the more stress response you exhibit. The belief that you have no power over your time or your environment is a leading cause of stress.

- Your environment has no predictability.
- You feel that your life circumstances are getting worse.

Once again, the issue in addressing chronic stress is not lack of information. It is a dissonant belief system that tells us that on the one hand we need to manage our stress, while insisting that we don't have time to invest in stress-reducing activities.

As discussed in previous chapters, we humans have three biological imperatives: survival, nourishment, and reproduction. These are hardwired to assure our survival as individuals and as a species. The stress response is one of the most powerful survival programs. It activates the sympathetic nervous system which then activates the pituitary and adrenal glands, increasing blood pressure and blood sugar, even suppressing the immune system. The stress response generates a battalion of steroids and peptides intended to divert all our resources to support the fight-or-flight response.

The biological arsenal meant to assure our escape from the saber-toothed tiger now keeps us at toxic stress levels. There is *no* physical threat to our survival. What triggers this stress mechanism is *our ability to visualize* worst-case scenarios, to imagine negative outcomes for future events. Think about it, our imagination has become a liability.

What is important is to understand is that we always have choices as to what *we make anything mean*. When our interpretation of events increases our stress level, we need to stop and ask: Why do I keep assigning this type of negative meaning to the events in my life? What would my wiser-self choose instead? What would I have to believe in order not to feel this stress?

Another major source of stress is our inability to relinquish control over the outcome of events. When we attempt to micro-manage everything, it taxes many of our resources. It also reflects our lack of trust and confidence in those around us. I have a friend whom I often drive to the airport. Whenever I call to ask what time she would like to be picked up it leads to a ten-minute discussion about the fourteen options that she needs to explore and the ramifications of each one. While on our way to the airport, she expresses her opinions about my driving speed, what lane I should be in – you get the picture, an extreme form of micro-management. Whenever others don't concur with her personal opinions, it generates a lot of stress for her – and when she is stressed, she eats. It is impossible for her to eat mindfully, because food is how she copes with stress, and as long as there are other people around, she is stressed out.

Most of us have heard Reinhold Niebuhr's famous quote. Once I accepted my complicity in how much stress I generated in my life, the following words took on a healing meaning:

Grant me the serenity to accept the things I cannot change,
The courage to change the things I can,
And the wisdom to know the *difference.*

Can you conceive of finding serenity, gratitude, and contentment in the midst of chaos and disappointment? Equanimity doesn't obliterate the tornado of our busy lives; instead it affords us the ability to go to the eye of the tornado. When we shift gears to become more detached or to recognize the gift in the situation before us, we acquire the ability to stress-proof our brains.

A stress-proof brain is maintained via healthy perspective, meaningful relationships, physical exercise, and mindfulness. We must deal with our challenges with wisdom, tenacity, joy, and gratitude. It is the ability to experience gladness, to leverage the resources available to us, and to feel grateful that stress-proofs our brains. It is being able to forgive when we are wronged. It is living in equanimity.

Here are some favorite quotes that have helped me stress-proof my brain:

May your own thoughts be gentle upon yourself. *Jonathan Lockwood Huie*

Who forces time is pushed back by time; who yields to time finds time on his side.
The Talmud

If your mind isn't clouded by unnecessary things, this is the best season of your life.
Wumen

Tools to Stress-Proof Our Brains

Let's take the ideas already presented and distill them into practical action.

Number 1 – Invest in a mindfulness practice. (And yes, I know, this is the one that causes the highest resistance, yet it has the highest pay off!)

Number 2 – Use aerobic exercise to dissipate the chemicals that your body generates to outrun the saber-toothed tiger. Your level of aerobic exertion should match your stress level.

Number 3 – Develop the habit of asking the questions: "What is the lesson that I could learn from this experience?" "What is the gift that is being offered to me?" "What keeps me from accepting it?"

Number 4 – Return to your body and to your environment every 15 minutes. Conscious breathing and noticing something new are the simplest ways to accomplish this objective.

Rewiring: How Long Will It Take?

There are five key factors that will determine how long it takes anyone to develop the necessary neural nets for a new skill, including the Naturally Thin Woman rewiring. These are:

1) An unconditional decision to restore healthy eating

2) The necessary time to re-establish nurturing behaviors

3) Maintaining a positive attitude while engaging in the rewiring activities

4) Resilience and tenacity to stay the course in the face of setbacks and

5) Acceptance of our humanity, that we are not perfect 100% of the time.

Factor 1 – Decide

Like so many of us I have lived through countless diets, and after most I experienced short periods of thinness. But deep down inside I was still a fat woman. Now I see that my weight had become the tangible evidence of my poor self-esteem. My overeating perpetuated the cycle of shame.

As a little girl I was not nurtured, which led me to believe that I was not special, I was never good enough. Every time I wanted to meet a man, every time I showed up for a new social event, every time I wanted to share an insight with anyone, the weight would drain my confidence. In my mind, I heard people saying, "If you're so smart, why are you so FAT?" I wanted desperately to return to my thin self, but I had not yet decided to stop the yo-yo dieting and find a comprehensive solution. Once I made that decision I was also able to stop feeding the cycle of shame. And until we decide to do whatever it takes to discover the source of our eating mania, we are doomed to bounce back and forth between the desire to be healthy and the seduction of the diets.

I'm reminded of a way you can tell whether a person has really given up smoking. They don't say, "I don't smoke;" they tell you emphatically, "I'm not a smoker." The distinction is profound. One states, "That is not an activity that I participate in" versus "I am not that type of person." One indicates a preference; the other is a declaration of personhood. To make a decision is to forfeit any other possibility. In fact, the Latin root of the word *decide* means "to cut off."

My transformational catharsis happened the day I DECIDED that come hell or high water I was stopping whatever was keeping me fat. That was the day that I divorced food as my lover, my energizer, my primary source of pleasure, and the one thing that I believed would make me feel better. Food no longer held the power it had over me, and that was the day that I decided to return to my naturally thin brain.

If, after you read this book, you resonate with its message and *decide* that you are ready to restore your THIN brain, you will invest in whatever is necessary to eradicate all of the beliefs and behaviors that keep you overeating. That decision will ensure that you stay on this journey, regardless of setbacks or challenges, as you uncover what truly feeds you. The strategies that will work for you are unique to your needs and personality. It is an excavation process, so be prepared for some trial and error. But know that your commitment to stay with this process for the long haul is critical. If all you are willing to do is "try it and see," the moment you encounter any potholes, detours, setbacks, or disappointments is the moment you will go off looking for another diet.

If the Thin Cognitive Behavior protocol speaks to your soul, DECIDE and promise yourself that whenever you experience a setback, you will take it as an opportunity to learn more about yourself, not as an excuse to give up on your personal journey.

Factor 2 – I Don't Have the Time!

Really? I discovered that the root cause of believing that I didn't have time was not recognizing that my anxiety level went through the roof every time I attempted to 1) do anything that required mindfulness, or 2) make my needs a priority. I felt antsy and restless whenever I tried to prepare a healthy meal to take to work, pack my yoga gear into my car, or turn off television in favor of an activity where I was required to be fully present. I used to call these activities "mindless tasks," as I honestly felt that they were beneath me, and I should not invest my time in them. I had better things to do. The mere idea of meditation triggered an anxiety attack.

What I didn't realize was that because of my high stress level I was not able to invest in anything that required presence and calmness. All I knew was the go-go, multi-task mantra of my society. I had to convince myself that the issue wasn't "I don't have time," but instead that the left side of my brain (which is the hemisphere that scheduled my day) would not agree to be muted for even a few minutes.

Yes, I know, we are all very busy; at one point I managed 45 people. But I personally know executives with thousands of people reporting to them who are effective precisely because they invest in a mindfulness practice. They exhibit the clarity to make difficult decisions and the uncanny ability to catch details that everyone else missed. These executives have experienced the return on their mindfulness investment as a pervasive sense of equanimity that translates into higher profits. So in fact, contrary to what most of us tell ourselves, we can't afford *not* to invest in a mindfulness practice.

Factor 3 – Positive Attitude

The single factor that has been scientifically documented to speed up the restoration of neural nets is how much pleasure (once again, alternative dopamine source) we experience while executing new behaviors. As early as 1996, when Dr. Schwartz developed the Cognitive Behavioral Therapy protocol, he noted that patients who felt enthusiastic and positive about the new therapy were the ones that rewired the quickest.

Rick Hanson, Ph.D., cofounder of the San Francisco Institute for Neuroscience and Contemplative Wisdom, explained that "stimulating areas of the brain that handle positive emotions strengthens those neural networks, just as working muscles strengthens them." The converse is also true, he explained. "If you routinely think about things that make you feel mad or wounded, you are sensitizing and strengthening the amygdala, which is primed to respond to negative experiences. So it will become more reactive, and you will get more upset more easily in the future."

One fascinating study documented that just by changing language from "I am fat" to "I currently carry more weight than I need," participants lost an average of eleven pounds! Eleven pounds, just by discharging this negative self-image that our weight is who we are! By rephrasing our self-concept from "I am" to "I currently carry," we cease to define our personhood in terms of weight.

Psychologists used to focus solely on the roots of why the mind *falters* – from mood disorders, anxiety, and depression to major psychotic illness. But in the past decade an increasing number of psychologists have been investigating what contributes to emotional *health*.

"We believe that a complete science and a complete practice of psychology should include an understanding of suffering and happiness, as well as their interaction, and validated interventions that both relieve suffering and increase happiness – two separate endeavors," wrote Martin Seligman, author of the books *Authentic Happiness* and *Learned Optimism* and Director of the University of Pennsylvania's Positive Psychology Center. Dr. Seligman was chosen as head of the American Psychological Association; his leadership catalyzed that group to study not just dysfunctions and illnesses but also the traits and characteristics of people who thrive. Seligman and colleagues came up with a handbook of characteristics to identify positive states of mind, as a parallel to psychiatry's "Diagnostic and Statistical Manual of Mental Disorders," the standard tool for diagnosing mental illness. Other psychologists devised happiness indexes and surveys to measure positive emotions.

More than 100 colleges and universities now offer classes in positive psychology, some of them teaching students not just the foundations but also how to apply the research to their personal lives. At Harvard University Tal Ben-Shahar's, Ph.D., lectures on positive psychology are the most popular classes on campus. Dr. Ben-Shahar's book *Being Happy: You Don't Have to Be Perfect to Lead a Richer, Happier Life* explains that the pursuit of perfection has negative impact on our quality of life. Sonja Lyubomirsky, Ph.D., a psychology professor at the University of California Riverside, is the author of *The How of Happiness*, a compilation of strategies and scientific research that can be used to increase happiness. "I've been studying this since my first day of graduate school," said Dr. Lyubomirsky, who remembers discussing the science of happiness with her adviser at Stanford. "At the time it was considered unscientific – soft and fuzzy – but now it's really hot."

One practice to return to a positive state of being is called Gratitude Intervention. Instead of relegating happiness to achieving some goal or acquiring a possession, Gratitude Intervention is the practice of acknowledging all of the people, events, and blessings, that we could be grateful for *today*. It has been noted that people who possess this ability experience a higher level of satisfaction than those who do not.

The point of this section is that how enthused you feel as you begin adopting the Naturally Thin Woman behaviors is what will determine if it's going to take weeks, months, or years to return to your Naturally Thin Woman neural nets! If you feel grateful, inspired, and motivated while performing the Naturally Thin Woman behaviors, it will take you a fraction of the time to restore the Naturally Thin Woman neural nets. However, if it is a chore and you have to push yourself to repeat these behaviors, propelled only by sheer willpower, or you feel drained or lack enthusiasm, it will take a lot longer. This is not a Pollyanna mentality, this is scientific fact: a positive, enthusiastic attitude shortens the rewiring process.

Factor 4 – Resilience and Tenacity

Resilience is the fourth most important success factor in restoring Naturally Thin Woman neural nets. The journey is an exploration and a return to our true essence. Tenacity is what allows us to accept that potholes and detours are part of the process. We might be disappointed during the journey but setbacks are part of arriving at the destination. Our unwavering determination, independent of how many obstacles we encounter, compels us to stay the course until we reach our goal.

For most of us, until we see the numbers on the scale heading down, we don't believe that the program is going to work. We must remember that our brain is currently wired to overeat, and that there are different triggers for different people: stress, emotional imbalance, and feeling socially uncomfortable are some examples. For others the trigger could be passing a bakery, or watching a commercial about a luscious piece of cheesecake.

Your experience with any type of movement might be non-existent. You may never have played any sports in school, you may never have felt a dopamine high after exercise, and your history could be devoid of the joy of team activities. Hence, food is your primary source for dopamine. Your upbringing could be laden with very specific foods, which now rekindle your sense of comfort, nurturing, and the joy of eating home cooking.

There is no such thing as failure, there are only setbacks. Every time we ignore our palate's signals that we are full, we must notice what led to that overindulgence. Every time we eat foods that don't contribute to our healing, we note the circumstances, people or emotions that contribute to our detours. Every time we don't invest the time to prepare a healthy meal, we review what exactly contributed to that decision.

To restore our naturally thin brain we must be willing to accept instances of setbacks and glean the positive information from that experience! Once we adopt that resiliency and tenacity we always succeed! One of my favorite quotes is by J. K. Rowling: "It is inevitable to live without failing at something. Unless you lived so cautiously you might as well not have lived at all. In which case, you fail by default."

Factor 5 – Plan to be Human

Accepting our humanity, including being overweight, contributes positively to our ability to eat mindfully. Kristin Neff, Ph.D., Professor at the University of Texas, did extensive research on the topic of self-compassion. Dr. Neff developed an empirical test that suggests that extending to *ourselves* the understanding and kindness that we typically extend only to *others* is a quality that contributes positively to our health. People who score high on Dr. Neff's self-compassion assessment typically experience less depression and anxiety, and tend to be happier and more optimistic.

One of my favorite quotes about this topic is by Pema Chödrön: "Compassionate action starts with seeing yourself when you start to make yourself right and when you start to make yourself wrong. At that point you could just contemplate the fact that there is a larger alternative to either of those, a more tender, shaky kind of place where you could live."

One of the concepts we touched upon in Chapter 2 is "ego depletion," that once we are emotionally *depleted* we are less likely to execute the activities that contribute to our well-being. We can compare our willpower to gas in a car: our internal drive/fortitude/energy is a limited resource, and it is used up during the day. As with a car, when we are driving around loaded down with a heavy cargo and making frequent stops, the gas will be used up more rapidly than during highway driving. Many successful people have accepted this fact, and that is why they invest in activities that contribute to them first thing in the morning, when the "ego is not depleted." Part of self-compassion, accepting our humanity, is to accept the limit of our resources and understand that once we reach that *EMPTY* mark on our personal gas gauge, our modest plans to execute the very things that contribute to us will be scuttled.

The knowledge that we possess precious, but limited, resources should not be used to beat ourselves up but instead to accept our humanity. The following are some examples that depict the effect of ego depletion in our lives:

- We are less likely to work out after having a challenging day.
- We are less likely to prepare a healthy meal when we get home after we gave it our all at the office.
- We are less likely to invest in activities for the next day – preparing meals, getting our workout gear packed – if we arrive at home emotionally exhausted.
- Our ability to select healthy, nutritious meals is compromised when we are dealing with high stress.
- Our resolution to eat less goes out the window after a fight with a family member.
- The likelihood of trusting our genuine appetite is jeopardized after seeing a disappointing number on the scale.
- We are less likely to execute healthy behaviors after a sleepless night.
- We have less patience with others after dealing with one difficult person.
- We experience emotional exhaustion after dealing with situations that require focused self-control.

As the adage goes, "Failure to plan is planning to fail." Accepting ego depletion is essential in planning a nurturing day. First and foremost we need to accept the fact that when we encounter demanding experiences, the rest of the day is compromised. Additionally, no perfect human being has ever existed; embracing this fact, as Dr. Neff has documented, is helpful. The best hitter in the entire history of baseball in his best season had a .440 average, which means that for every 10 times he went to bat, he was out 6 times!

It is vital to recognize our human needs: love and belonging, earning respect, being recognized, unadulterated enjoyment, laugher, learning, change, relaxation, choice and independence. Knowing these, we need to be aware of how, when and where we can refuel. How do we replenish our stamina? Do we schedule treats just because? Can we distinguish between *yum* experiences and *yuck* experiences? What truly restores us after a challenging day? Should we go for a brisk walk/run before continuing our day running on fumes? If we are completely spent after work, should we schedule a massage? Meditate? Watch an uplifting movie? Take a soothing bath? Read a good book? Indulge in joyful movement? Make a phone call to a nurturing friend? What can we plan that is restorative after being completely depleted? So instead of getting food from the most convenient drive-through, can we anticipate those types of days and have a convenient healthy meal identified? And yes, in some instances the wiser course, the most effective, loving thing we can do for ourselves is to veg and restore.

Chapter 9 Summary

When you do decide that this program is what will help you once and for all to restore your healthy brain, as with any long journey, the more prepared you are, the higher the likelihood of success.

A commitment to invest time in activities that nurture you, that improve the quality of your life is necessary. Scientists have been documenting the power of positive thinking. By leveraging a positive attitude you can significantly shorten the time that it takes to restore your Naturally Thin Woman neural nets.

Resilience and tenacity are important on this journey home. Self-compassion is also a contributing factor in achieving success.

One final tip I suggest is to make a serious commitment to stress-proof your brain. Most stress today comes from our own minds, not from the exterior world. That means we can manage our stress levels by changing our minds! When we invest in healthy outlets for what is truly stressing us, our quality of work and life improves. Don't forget, it's a process. By using strategies like meditation or frequent mindful moments, we can achieve the state of equanimity needed to succeed in the Naturally Thin Woman program. Take stock of what works for you personally. What worked for me may not work in the same manner for you. That's what our website is for, to get you through the bumps in the road. This is not a one-size-fits-all program. It is a program about getting in touch with your needs.

Chapter 10 – Implementing THE Program

Exile the Scale

Before we begin, there is a requirement that might push all of your emotional buttons: you will need to throw away your scale. Yes. To begin the program, record your measurements and your initial weight as your starting point, but then exile the scale to an inaccessible location, preferably Tierra del Fuego.

You are embarking on a voyage back to your core essence, a journey reinstating your inner wisdom, the state of being where you are going to reclaim trust in your appetite. Your body will go through adaptive phases, perhaps even *gain* a few pounds, before it settles into the rhythm of consistent weight loss.

The issue is that on days when the scale goes up, it jeopardizes your ability to listen to your authentic wisdom, because you feel demoralized. Suddenly, all of that effort feels like a waste of time and, before you know it, you are emotionally in need of some solace and probably looking for that box of Ding Dongs®. The days that the scale ekes down, we overanalyze what we ate the previous day and begin plotting to replicate it. Neither of these strategies contributes to being present to your palate in order to use it as the barometer of hunger and satiation. That background noise is detrimental to listening to your inner voice, to that wisdom that will tell you when you are full, that will restore your trust in your own physical hunger. It is vitally important to measure progress, but the scale is simply not reliable, as water retention, set point, and hormonal changes all influence that number.

Secondly, we have been socialized to keep looking at the scale for validation, for evidence of beauty and worth. Yes, we do want to experience progress, but we must measure it by better standards. Our focus is on inner guidance, that internal voice that differentiates between physical hunger and brain hunger. From the perspective of lifelong change, ending the cycle of external validation is critical.

Step 4 is to experience progress in how you *feel*. Do you know how amazing it feels to look at a plate full of food and say to yourself, "I've had enough. I'm not hungry. I don't need to clear the plate." When you give your power to an external device, like the scale, you compromise the opportunity to reconnect to what really feeds you, the trust that keeps you naturally thin. Is it more important that the scale reflect a specific number or that you eradicate overeating, binges, and mindless snacks and restore the genuine pleasure of eating?

Profound changes happen over a matter of weeks, not from one day to another. This is a lifelong relationship, not a one-night stand. A meaningful checkpoint is six weeks after starting the program, when you have experienced amazing progress in the stages we will identify here. Give yourself time to make the significant progress that will restore your Naturally Thin Woman neural nets.

The program will ask you to track progress in a number of areas that will increase your self-esteem, energy level, trust in yourself, and genuine appetite. Once you have restored your Naturally Thin Woman brain, you will be astounded. You will be attuned to your inner frequency, you will be renewed, and you will reconnect to something more profound than a number on a scale.

The Thin Woman's Brain

We'll finish this section about exiling the scale with a quote by T.D. Jakes: "When you hold on to your history, you do it at the expense of your destiny."

Stage 1 – Mindfulness and Hunger Recognition

We first described mindfulness in Chapter 3 and then devoted the entirety of Chapter 5 to this subject. We outlined many options for a mindfulness practice. One of these options was a mindful moment where you can take three deep breaths, which facilitates reconnecting to your body. Once you are fully present to your body, notice something new; this will allow you to be present to your environment. During the prerelease trial of this book, we discovered that what most busy women find easiest is 25 mindful moments per day. It is now time to begin your chosen mindfulness practice.

I'm a huge advocate of meditation, a practice that has many benefits. It has been demonstrated to increase the blood flow to your prefrontal cortex, the part of the brain associated with mindfulness. In fact, entire books have been written on the subject of meditation, and it is actually quite simple:

a) Secure a place where you will not be disturbed.
b) Turn off all potential distractions: phone, computer, etc.
c) Sit comfortably, upright, feet on the floor.
d) Take deep breaths.
e) Focus 100% of your attention on your breath.
f) Whenever your mind wanders off, gently bring it back to your breath.

That's it! No esoteric mumbo-jumbo, no mysticism. Just focus on your breath and return your attention to it whenever your mind wanders off. Do not be overly concerned about how many times your mind detours, especially at the beginning; it doesn't matter. It's the act of bringing your focus back to the breath that builds your mindfulness "muscles." The more times you do it, the more natural and easy it becomes. Don't beat yourself up if you don't "get it" right away. Keep practicing – you will!

Because your brain is currently food-obsessed, it is highly probable that you are constantly thinking about food and are always brain-hungry. "Am I physically hungry?" This will become your mantra during Stage 1. Just make sure that you have your checklist from Chapter 3 ready: Is my stomach growling? Is my blood-sugar level low? Do I have any evidence of physical hunger?

When you are a food addict, your mouth will water at the slightest external stimulus, what we call "social, sensual, thought, physiological and emotional triggers," as discussed in Chapter 3. Just remember, mouthwatering is *not* exclusive to physical hunger; food addicts also experience it when faced with a food trigger.

Stage 1 Measure of Success: When you are able to experience 25 mindful moments per day AND you are able to differentiate between brain hunger and physical hunger for at least four consecutive days, you are ready to move to Stage 2!

Please note: What is necessary to advance to Stage 2 is that you can concretely demonstrate that you are successful with these two objectives. We are not proposing you just *attempt* these objectives for four days; we are encouraging you to be honest with yourself and to remain in Stage 1 until you are able to experience *success* with these two objectives for at least four consecutive days. Remember, you are rewiring your brain; a strong foundation is what will support you in being successful during this journey.

Stage 2 – TCB Protocol for Easy Food Triggers

During Stage 2 you continue investing in your mindfulness practice. In Stage 1, if you started meditating and you were able to do 10 minutes per sitting, increase it to 15 minutes. If you were able to do 25 mindful moments, do 30.

Now that you are able to reliably execute *Step 1: Recognize Brain Hunger*, you are ready to start Steps 2 through 4 of the TCB protocol when dealing with *easy* food triggers.

> Step 2: Observe the brain hunger
> Step 3: Name the real need and address it
> Step 4: Measure progress and experience success

Remember that we included three powerful tools (EMDR, EFT and NLP Anchors) in Chapter 6 to help you deal with Step 2. These tools are especially helpful if your food addiction score is SEVERE.

As described in Chapter 4, there are many types of triggers that cause brain hunger. You will find *Step 3: Name the real need and address it* will be easiest with triggers that don't push your limits. Most women find it straightforward to recognize "sensual, thought, and physiological" triggers. Many that are extroverted tend to feel comfortable in social environments and typically don't experience a significant amount of anxiety when addressing social triggers. However, if you have a history of social anxiety, dealing with social triggers might be more challenging. Categorically, we are going to call any food triggers that are manageable for you "easy food triggers": easy for you to *name the real need* and where you can readily *address the real need*. Some examples of being able to execute Step 3 for easy food triggers are:

- In the past the only way you stopped working was by eating something; now you recognize the brain hunger as your body telling you that you need a break.
- You recognize that you were not hungry before the opportunistic food cue: seeing a food commercial or passing by a bakery or being offered food at work. Now you are able to name your "hunger" as your automatic reaction to food exposure. You walk away from the food commercial or the bakery without any trauma or anxiety. When offered food, you are able to express appreciation for the gesture and return to your day serenely.

All of these types of sensual triggers are within your comfort level. In Stage 2, we are looking for progress with all of the food triggers within your emotional capacity.

Stage 2 Measure of Success – You experience success with these *easy food triggers*. Of equal importance is to recognize and document any areas where you were not able to name the real need or were simply at a loss as to why you could not identify it. In other instances, you could name the real need but you may have not been able to address it.

If you are able to execute all four steps of the TCB protocol for *easy food triggers*, those within your emotional capacity, without struggle or anxiety for four consecutive days, you are now ready to move on to Stage 3.

Stage 3 – Eating Mindfully at Home*

Remember to continue investing in your mindfulness practice. Follow the process outlined in Chapter 5 and eat mindfully at home.

*The assumption is that home is your most tranquil atmosphere; however, if home is chaotic, identify an alternative setting that allows you to eat mindfully.

Stage 3 Measure of Success: You are able to eat mindfully at home (or in your most tranquil environment) for at least four consecutive days – or until you are confident that you are ready to move on to the next stage. Do not worry, this is not a race. Be consistent, leverage your wisdom, think long-term. The tortoise always gets to the finish line before the rabbit.

Stage 4 – Reintroducing Forbidden Foods

Keep investing in your mindfulness practice. Take it to the next level.

Now that you have proven success with *Stage 3: Eat Mindfully at Home*, pick the one food you don't even allow yourself to keep in the house, because whenever you attempt to eat it you basically have a binge. For some women, it's rich, creamy ice cream; for others it is gooey pastries, or pizza, or nachos. What is *your* forbidden food? What is the one food that you don't trust yourself to eat because once you start you can't stop? What is the one food that you simply can't eat in reasonable amounts?

For Stage 4 of the rewiring, you must eat that forbidden food in a mindful manner. You will eat it every single day until your brain learns that you can experience satisfaction eating a single serving of that food when you eat it *mindfully*. Now let's clarify what a small amount is:

- Rich creamy ice cream: one scoop, not one scoop that looks like two, but one scoop
- Gooey pastry: half a pastry, and not from one pastry that looks like a pie
- Rich and creamy chocolate: two small pieces
- Pizza: one slice
- Nachos: two ounces (use a kitchen scale)

When in doubt, read what is considered one serving and actually eat that amount. Using your emerging mindfulness, you will be astonished when you experience genuine satisfaction with only one serving of your forbidden food.

Please remember that flavor-enhanced foods are addicting. Any food with extra sugar, extra salt, or any of the chemical enhancers, such as MSG, directly stimulates the pleasure center of the brain. Once this center is stimulated, you'll have a difficult time being able to recognize satiation.

Stage 4 Measure of Success – You are able to experience genuine satisfaction after mindfully eating one small serving of your forbidden food for at least four consecutive days, or until you are confident that you are ready to move on to the next stage. Remember, you are rewiring your brain. Embrace the long-term perspective; you want a foundation that is solid and strong.

Stage 5 – Eating Mindfully in a Challenging Environment

You now have experienced success in your ability to identify brain hunger and execute the entire TCB protocol. You also know that you can eat mindfully in your most tranquil environment, and you are able to eat what were previously labeled forbidden foods and experience satisfaction by eating just one serving. Hooray!

Let's take these emerging Naturally Thin Woman neural nets to the next level. Your continued investment in your mindfulness practice is really going to pay off in Stage 5. For some women it is more challenging to eat mindfully with their families (as home is a chaotic environment). For others, the challenge is eating with their in-laws or at a large party. You fill in the specifics: what is a challenging eating environment for you?

It is now time to raise the bar. This should not be your most daunting eating environment, but it should be a setting requiring more emotional resources than eating in a tranquil environment.

In order to be successful in challenging environments, many of us need to leverage tools that allow us to remain connected to our bodies – tools such as conscious breathing, EMDR, and many others – any practice that supports your ability to experience emotional imbalance with equanimity.

Stage 5 Measure of Success – You feel the "brain hunger" overwhelming you, but you are able to observe and interrupt the food fantasy and name which emotional buttons are being pushed. You are able to address the real need: You want the loud TV off! You need the children to stop screaming! You're sick of the family fights! External challenges that typically initiated the "stuff my face" programing are now recognized. You are able to *name the real need and address it* without blindly executing the old overeating program.

Instead of resorting to your old behavior of shoveling food, you self-soothe and eat mindfully. This is tremendous progress. You were pushed to your limit but you were able to interrupt the brain hunger, give it a name, and address what needed to be fed. Again, recognize the progress; you name your need instead of mindlessly eating as you did in the past. When you are able to successfully experience four instances of eating mindfully in a challenging environment, you are well on your way to restoring your Naturally Thin Woman neural nets.

Stage 6 – TCB for Moderate Food Triggers

Humans are pleasure-seeking beings. All addicts seek a dopamine high when they experience emotional discomfort. Because our brains have been hard-wired to associate pleasure with food, anything that causes us emotional discomfort will trigger brain hunger.

At the beginning of the TCB process, when we attempt to recognize any emotion that has been deeply socialized as *not OK*, we might have difficulty naming it. Some of these triggers must not only be named but also may require resources not yet in our emotional toolbox. Stress cannot be intellectualized; it must be managed through significant action, as described in Chapter 9. Understanding our inability to express anger will not make it go away. We need to learn how to pour that anger onto paper or express it fully in a physical manner (some women find a punching bag helpful). We might also seek help from a friend. Just knowing that you experience brain hunger when you return to your empty house will not end the emotional eating. The change comes from converting your home into your place of refuge and comfort, as these are effective steps to address your real needs.

The point is that in order to make progress in this stage of the rewiring, many women have to invest time and effort developing new skills to address their real needs. For example, suppose that you find yourself in an unreasonable work environment where you are frequently expected to give up your weekends. However, you lack the confidence to stand up for yourself and the negotiation skills to convince your boss that better planning is necessary. As a prudent step you also want to polish your computer skills and update your resume, as that will give you the self-assurance to take these steps.

Prior to beginning this process, you were unable to name what was triggering your sudden hunger. But now you recognize that every time the boss asks you to give up your weekend, you experience disappointment, rage, and hopelessness. It is the first time that you have given your feelings a name.

You now understand your internal process. You haven't magically acquired the skills to address your needs, but you now appreciate the investment needed to eradicate the root cause of your overeating behavior. And yes, some of these changes are not overnight fixes but they are extremely worthwhile, as they contribute to your growth.

You can find many tools to deal with emotional eating in Appendix A.

Stage 6 Measure of Success – You are able to name difficult emotional triggers that in the past blindly led you to overeat. You are willing to name whatever shame caused you to suppress your personal needs. You take meaningful action in obtaining the tools – conscious breathing, self-advocacy, permission to experience rage – that allow you to address the real need. In some instances professional support is helpful for developing the tools we need to stand up for ourselves.

Stage 7 – TCB Protocol for Overwhelming Triggers

Let me emphasize that not everyone has difficulty identifying food triggers. However, if you find yourself in a recurrent pattern where you experience "I know that I am not physically hungry, but I can't identify why I still want to overeat," then a deeper excavation is merited. We must understand that, at a fundamental level, all addictive behaviors return us to the cycle of shame. For a food addict, the most tangible example of the cycle of shame is how we feel after a binge: "I did it again. How could I have eaten all of that food? I feel awful. I feel beaten. I am so worthless, such a loser, such a *fat* woman!" Sometimes our inability to address whatever is masquerading as hunger is our inability to dismantle our belief system. But let me repeat that when one of our core beliefs is that we are flawed, anything that causes us to feel inadequate will continue expressing itself as hunger.

You must be willing to embrace your humanity and take advantage of any tool that allows you to face the cycle of shame. There are many aids that can be leveraged during this stage: journaling, expressing your needs to a helpful friend, researching the specific issue that fuels your emotional hunger, participating in a seminar on the topic, or seeking professional help. Appendix A is wholly dedicated to the topic of emotional hunger.

Stage 7 Measure of Success – You recognize your most challenging food triggers. You understand that your addiction could be to the cycle of shame. You are able to name painful food triggers. You take meaningful action in leveraging the tools available, establishing self-advocacy, and if necessary, working with professionals – all of which allow you to address the real needs that fuel a hunger caused by overwhelming emotional triggers. You are finally able to address your needs instead of eating through them.

Stage 8 – Eating Mindfully in a Daunting Situation

For many years I heard about the Harvard study of what people fear most: public speaking came in first, death second. Jerry Seinfeld once quipped, "So, if you're at a funeral, you'd rather be the guy in the casket than the one delivering the eulogy." While this is not true across the board, most people experience some level of anxiety with anything that is outside their comfort zone. If the experience is *far* outside of your comfort zone, it can lead to unbearable distress, which for a food addict results in overeating. The normal human reaction is to try to find comfort as quickly as possible. Food is easily accessible; it is cheap, legal and pleasurable. Eating is the logical reaction for anyone who primarily associates relief with food. The moment that we food addicts face a daunting situation, we experience hunger. Obviously, once we experience that non-food options are more soothing, we can leverage these healthy alternatives. However, if all we find soothing is food, the brain will always go to whatever makes us feel good, and the quicker the better.

Any emotion that contradicts our mental stories might be repressed (please refer to *Appendix A – The Truth Will Make You Hungry*). Note the environments, people, and situations that trigger daunting brain hunger. If you don't have a clear idea of what exactly is fueling your overeating behavior, understanding, perhaps researching, why people repress their emotions might be necessary. If you can get through Steps 1 and 2 but continue to experience inexplicable hunger, then you might benefit from working with a professional who has expertise in releasing repressed emotions and who could help you address whatever you are repressing.

Stage 8 Measure of Success – You are aware of situations, people or environments way outside your comfort zone. You might need to develop effective coping mechanisms to deal with them. In some cases, identifying and accepting repressed emotions and releasing the story that kept them repressed will mark the end of your unconscious eating.

Stage 9 – Establish the Roots of a Weed

Did you know that some diet shakes do help some people lose 8 pounds in one week? Yes, for some people carrying a lot of extra water, it does happen. And yes, building a house on a mudslide-prone hill takes less time when they skip the structural support that ensures stability. But you know what happens to those houses when there is the slightest environmental challenge.

Some women begin experiencing positive results within weeks of starting the Naturally Thin Woman program, and it's wonderful. It allows them to experience success and freedom, which ensures that they keep on going. One of the errors in restoring neural nets is to count your chickens before they're hatched – to assume the wiring is complete when you've reached your ideal dress size. But by now you know that the speediest path is not always what results in lifelong rewiring. So while being able to systematically go through the TCB protocol and learning to eat mindfully are necessary stages, they don't represent the completion of the rewiring.

The maintenance phase of our Naturally Thin Woman program takes place during that critical first year after achieving a healthy weight. Case studies of addicts have taught us that we should plan to remain attentive *for at least one year* to ensure that our neural nets get irreversibly restored.

When food addicts are only given a set of coping tools while the brain remains addicted to food, they are perennially susceptible to relapses, always at the mercy of potential food triggers. That is why the solution is to rewire the brain out of its addiction and restore it to its healthy, pre-addiction state. That is the key difference between the Naturally Thin Woman program and accumulating a bunch of eating strategies that do not eradicate the addictive behavior.

You may ask why we want to continue the TCB process for a full year. Did you know that some bamboo can grow up to ten feet per day? However, when we look at that bamboo's root system, it is shallow and weak. If a tornado hits a bamboo plant, it is gone. In contrast, the root system of a weed is deeper, wider and stronger. If a weed is hit, its complex, fibrous root system allows it to restore itself. We must strive to build neural nets so strong that they can withstand any life challenge without returning us to overeating as a coping mechanism. The prayer goes, "Lord, give me the tenacity of a weed, and remind me that nothing is impossible."

Stage 9 Measure of Success – Your immediate reactions to difficult challenges, emotional discomfort, unexpected setbacks, profound disappointment – the ups and downs of life – have been replaced with life-enhancing and nurturing options. Examples of these coping mechanisms include deep breathing, journaling, counseling, punching a bag, calling a friend, and/or moderate to vigorous exercise. You genuinely feel that these alternatives are more helpful than eating; your brain no longer fantasizes about food the moment that you face challenges.

It is highly recommended to execute the TCB protocol and eat mindfully for an entire year after reaching your desired dress size. This is a precautionary measure to ensure that your roots, your Naturally Thin Woman neural nets, are as strong as the roots of a weed. You are changing your biology, not just acquiring habits, and your new brain wiring must be healthy enough to function not only when everything is manageable, but also when life presents you with overwhelming challenges.

Stage 10 – Returning to Eating Naturally

The signs that your Naturally Thin Woman neural nets have been restored are many:

- You no longer salivate at the mere sight of food cues, such as TV commercials, magazine photographs, and the cake or bread aisle at the supermarket. Physiologically, the Pavlovian response is gone.
- You no longer daydream about food.
- Only physical hunger leads you to begin the process of "What do I want to eat? What am I truly hungry for? What is my body asking for?"
- You eat mindfully; the days of shoveling food as quickly as humanly possible are gone.
- It doesn't matter how much food remains on the plate, you trust that when the food loses its taste, your body is telling you that it is satisfied.
- Instances of brain hunger are rare, in fact almost non-existent. But if they do occur, you recognize them immediately, and you can address the underlying need.
- You are able to experience life's ups and downs without resorting to overeating, as you now accept that overeating feeds the cycle of shame.
- The overwhelming power that food had over you is completely gone.
- You are no longer a food addict. You are no longer at the mercy of your food obsessions.
- Sharing a meal is not the only avenue to spending quality time with friends.
- Overeating anxieties are completely gone, and you can experience genuine satisfaction eating in a mindful manner.
- You experience the freedom of trusting your palate.
- There are no forbidden foods. Once you are physically hungry, you trust your body's messages as to what it needs.
- You are now able to experience genuine satisfaction when eating mindfully, and small amounts are honest-to-goodness satisfying.
- You continue to invest in the life tools that allow you to foster self-advocacy and self-knowledge.
- You experience freedom. You have reclaimed your ability to select foods that sound good without any fear that you will gain weight.
- Eating has ceased to be hazardous to your psyche; eating is now a pleasure. The fear that you might overeat is completely gone.
- The kitchen ceases to be a hostile environment, and you can actually reclaim the joy of cooking.
- You are now free from the tyranny of diets, reinstating your trust in what nourishes you, re-establishing a healthy dopamine level.
- Finally, your Naturally Thin Woman neural nets have been restored!

Contrary to popular belief, eating mindfully, regardless of *what* you are eating, actually allows your body to release the extra fat! Why? You are naturally eating a fraction of the amount that you used to *over*eat mindlessly. There is no diet book telling you what or how much you should be eating. Instead you are now paying attention to your body's inner guidance. You have learned to trust your body's signals. It doesn't want pizza and ice cream every single day; it will naturally hunger for nourishing, life-sustaining foods.

When we learn to eat mindfully, food stops hijacking our brain into overeating and bingeing; we automatically consume fewer calories, because that's what feels natural. This eating process is one that is directed by your self-advocacy and self-knowledge – your Naturally Thin neural nets, which don't count calories, yet keep you from overeating because it no longer feels good.

Stage 10 Measure of Success – Once we are responding to genuine hunger and eating what truly nourishes us, something truly magical happens. Our body's messages become clearer, and we know that this wisdom will return us to a healthy balance. No longer do we muffle our inner voice in favor of a diet that, in the long run, is counter to our own best interests.

After just a few weeks following the TCB protocol, most women experience feeling truly free; for many, it is the first time in years. All of the energy wasted beating ourselves up – the toxic inner dialogue when we deviate from the diet, how we were not supposed to eat this, how much we overate of that – all of that squandered life force is returned to us.

Restoring your thin woman's brain is an amazing achievement. Celebrate it! You have reclaimed your life!

Possible Challenges Summarized

This section summarizes potential challenges that might arise as you undertake the Naturally Thin Woman program. Awareness of pitfalls is always helpful so that they won't derail us as we embark on the process.

Objective	Possible Challenges
Throwing away the scale **Evidence of Restoring NTW Neural Nets** • You relearn how genuine fullness feels in your body. You trust that your body's messages are more important than any external device. • When you do weigh yourself, you remember that the number you see is affected by many factors, and it doesn't always reflect your progress.	You feel terrified that if you don't rely on a scale, you will gain weight. External validation is more important than your own body awareness.
Willingness to label your hunger triggers	• Awkwardness when you begin to

Objective	Possible Challenges
and to go through the four steps of the TCB protocol **Evidence of Restoring NTW Neural Nets** • The compulsive, overwhelming power that food has over you begins to subside.	execute the TCB protocol; it might feel too foreign. • Inability to recognize the difference between the two types of hunger, which is a function of self-awareness. • If the levels of addiction or stress are very high, the first step, "Recognize Brain Hunger" might require a substantial investment in a mindfulness practice before developing this capacity.
Eating only when you are physically hungry **Evidence of Restoring NTW Neural Nets** • You are no longer at the mercy of obsessive and compulsive food attacks.	• But I am always hungry! • Developing the ability to go through the "Do I have any evidence of physical hunger" check list and accumulate tangible evidence that your body is experiencing physical hunger. • Unwillingness to identify what is asking for attention. • Learning to self-soothe, or having the personal resources to help you work through your emotional needs. • Having the courage to address the need.
Eating Mindfully **Evidence of Restoring NTW Neural Nets** The anxiety vanishes and you experience genuine satisfaction when eating in a mindful manner.	• If your food addiction score is SEVERE waiting to eat until the food gets on the table might generates stratospheric anxiety. You literally can't keep yourself from eating in the kitchen or directly from the refrigerator.
Reintroducing forbidden foods into your diet **Evidence of Restoring NTW Neural Nets** • Experiencing a sense of freedom; you feel genuine satisfaction when mindfully eating small amounts of these forbidden foods.	• Incredulity and tangible fear (I will eat the entire pizza, the entire tub of ice cream, the entire bag of nacho chips, all of the chocolate, at least six Danishes). • A lack of trust that your body will know when it's satisfied. • Until you experience the benefit of this process, you might experience high levels of anxiety.
After you've learned to eat mindfully,	- Noticeable fear: I'm going to

Objective	Possible Challenges
trusting your taste buds and allowing yourself to eat whatever you want **Evidence of Restoring NTW Neural Nets** • A feeling of freedom; for the first time in years you can trust your ability to select foods based on your body's needs.	blow up like a puffer fish.
Reclaiming a genuine joy of eating, and for some, the joy of cooking! **Evidence of Restoring NTW Neural Nets** • Eating stops being a crap shoot. You stop worrying whether you are going to binge or eat within the constraints of your current diet. • Freedom from the tyranny of diets, reinstatement of your ability to eat mindfully, repairing a healthy dopamine level.	- Trusting that you can enjoy food and return to natural thinness - For many women changing the belief that "I don't have time to shop, cook, and clean"

Throughout the book we have included a variety of tools to support you during your journey. The most important are: a mindfulness practice and the five factors described earlier in this chapter as necessary for your success. Many people who pursue CBT based programs do so with the guidance of a clinician or therapist, for those wanting or needing additional support, we offer a variety of programs and tools including a smart device APP. For additional information please visit www.thinwomanbrain.com.

In Appendix B we address special cases that might be applicable if you can't measure tangible success after three weeks of consistently executing the Naturally Thin Woman program.

The Invitation

It is my profound privilege to invite you to be fully present to your own life. You no longer have to live at the mercy of a food-obsessed brain; you no longer need to invest Herculean efforts to perpetuate a diet lifestyle. The Naturally Thin Woman program, at its core, is about reconnecting with your inner wisdom. All the time and energy that you used to invest in dieting and self-loathing are now returned to you. It is up to you to reinvest them creatively on your personal growth, your family, your community, and your passions.

This is the time to ask yourself what is beckoning you to become the leading lady in your own life. Who do you want to be, and what are you willing to invest in order to become that woman?

The tools presented in this book will help you establish a healthy relationship with food. By repeating the TCB steps and mindful eating, you will come to trust your inner guidance. This is an opportunity to know yourself intimately and to become your most ardent advocate. What would you dare to dream if you knew that finally you could end the dieting cycle and live the life that you were meant to live? All you have to do is accept this invitation.

Chapter 10 Summary

You may be feeling a bit overwhelmed at the moment. You just absorbed a lot of information. If you feel that way, it's okay! Luckily, Chapter 10 breaks down the process into stages that insure success. You don't have to achieve all of the objectives all at once, just tackle one stage at a time until you experience success.

This program is not something that you can commit to halfway and still expect to return to eating like a Naturally Thin Woman. If these concepts speak to you, you must commit yourself wholeheartedly, and your investment will eradicate overeating once and for all.

Epilogue

One of the women who participated in the prerelease trial of this book, after experiencing the magnificent freedom to trust herself and eat whatever sounded appealing to her, asked me to include this short poem titled, *"When Was the Last Time?"* It is a piece I wrote as an expression of our longings, what we yearn for when we experience emotional hunger.

When was the last time that you ...

- Wrote your name on the sand?

- Wondered where exactly is Timbuktu?

- Witnessed a death (of a relationship, a marriage, a dream)?

- Watched the children play?

- Talked for two hours in bed?

- Swung so high that you could touch eternity?

- Shared a champagne picnic?

- Laughed until your belly hurt?

- Held your dream within the clouds?

- Saw a universe in a grain of sand?

- Felt like the best version of yourself?

- Experienced sunrise?

- Embraced someone's pain?

- Danced until you sweated ... and didn't notice it?

- Cried with someone else?

- Climbed to the top of the mountain?

- Celebrated someone else's essence?

- Built a sand sculpture?

- Brought someone breakfast in bed?

When was the last time you felt truly present to life? When was the last time you loved yourself?

Appendix A – The Truth Will ... Make You Hungry

The intent of this addendum is to shed light, using personal examples, on those women whose overeating behaviors stem from emotional issues. If you feel that emotional overeating is not your issue, you might want to skip this addendum. For those who know that emotional imbalance is their primary trigger to overeat, please note that there are hundreds upon hundreds of books dedicated to this topic. However, when you are physically addicted to food, rewiring your brain back to health is critical. Think about it, even if you learn how to address your emotional needs, if you are physiologically addicted to food, you will continue to have physical cravings.

Most human beings, when confronted with difficult people, challenging situations, or stressful environments, experience "ego depletion" (a concept introduced in Chapter 2) and try to restore their sense of well-being as quickly and easily as possible. For most addicts, that translates into seeking solace in their drug of choice, for two very important reasons:

1. When we lack the personal tools and/or support to deal effectively with these human emotions, our only choice is to avoid them.
2. The brain associates pleasure with the drug; hence it is perceived as a way of forgetting the "bad day."

During the many years of my quest to lose weight, I accumulated a stack of "human potential" and self-help books where others shared their issues, traumas, and how they used food to suppress their emotions. I literally could not read these stories. The first hint that I might have to examine my past or recognize my own needs sent the book into the recycling bin. At this time I was a single mother, holding a demanding corporate job, with no financial support from my ex. I simply did not have the bandwidth to work on personal growth – or at least that's the story I was telling myself.

I wasn't interested in things that required introspection or profound changes. I was, however, very interested in anything in the form of a diet, pill, or exercise program. At that time I didn't know which events caused my lack of body awareness, and I didn't realize that there was such a thing as emotional hunger. Because I had not developed confidence or self-advocacy, food was how I dealt with any imbalance in my life.

I did not possess the inner resources that allowed me to accept my humanity. Instead I bolstered an idealized identity – my effervescent personality – to hide my vulnerability. Any emotional disturbance would send me to the refrigerator faster than a new millionaire could acquire friends.

What is the source of our inability to be truthful with ourselves? What is the fear that we harbor in the cave of our subconscious? Why do we stuff our feelings instead of honoring our humanity? Why can't we accept that we are as flawed as the next person? Where did we learn to suppress so many emotions?

In order to answer some of these questions, let's first look at the difference between suppression and repression.

Suppression is a conscious choice not to indulge a particular thought, feeling, or action. We are *aware* of a thought or feeling, but we decide not to *dwell* on it (internally, by continuing to think about it) – nor to *express* it (externally, by acting out). Usually we suppress emotions because we believe that it is inappropriate to deal with them at the moment. Suppression is a useful psychological mechanism that permits us to concentrate on our affairs without being distracted by every impulse that arises.

Repression is similar to suppression – it is a thought, feeling, or emotion that is not expressed, but in repression, we deny that the element even exists. We reject these feelings because our innate self-protection mechanism (usually unconscious) blocks them so they will not disrupt our psychological stability. But stability and self-image that are based on rejection of reality are no more than illusions.

When we don't have the ability to face emotional challenges and instead we repress them with food, our brain becomes wired to label emotional distress as *hunger.*

Repression Mechanism

The ability to identify what is fueling "emotional hunger" is based on an awareness of our belief systems and values. The capacity to effectively deal with these root causes is a function of our courage to face unreleased traumas and accept our humanity. Many of us have mental stories (repressions) that don't allow us to see what lies behind the emotional hunger, such as:

- An idealized childhood, when in fact the truth would shatter family relationships
- A fairy tale of a happy marriage, when in fact there are emotional issues that threaten its stability
- The prestige of a prominent profession, when in fact the work is not our life's passion and staying in the job perpetuates overwhelming stress
- The privileges of a prosperous life with hundreds of acquaintances but no genuine friends
- Letting our achievements hide the fact that our life has no meaning or purpose
- Extolling the joys of motherhood when in fact we feel trapped with our preschoolers.

Our ability to identify anything threatening the current status quo is part of the "name and address the real need" step. My own personal story is that of a neglected child. However, I was unwilling to accept that plot line, as it would have desecrated the shrine that I had erected to my dad, a man who had died suddenly at 43. Another story was my over-identification with the prestigious, world-class consulting engagements that consumed 80 hours of every week. Then there was me as a young mother, abandoned by my husband when our son was barely five months old. I was unable to face the anguish, betrayal, and depression that scarred my psyche.

So yes, I lived these stories, and I now understand how I repressed them. If your repression mechanism is deeply entrenched, just reading these passages might not afford you the certitude and/or courage to face what is fueling your own emotional hunger. The paradox is that avoiding the fear feeds it – in the case of emotional hunger, literally!

There is a wide spectrum of human issues that manifest as emotional eating. Food is just the symptom; food is just your repression mechanism. It is outside the scope of this book to address every possible human psychological need. The important thing is to be able to recognize when the "Measure Your Progress" step is completely stalled, because there might be repressed emotions that need to be addressed. If that is the case, you owe it to yourself to have the courage to ask:

- Do I truly like/love myself?
- Do I feel worthwhile as a human being?
- Do I have supportive friendships, meaningful work, a loving family, and nurturing self-advocacy?
- Is it possible that food is how I avoid facing my problems?

Eating for most of us is not about nutrition. It is about calming our nervous system when we get stressed out. It is about experiencing pseudo-release when we are ready to explode. It is returning to an empty house and attempting to capture a sense of "home" via food. It is a Pavlovian response where specific activities, such as watching TV, are coupled with eating. It is about being part of a social community where we express love with food. It is about believing that food is going to make us feel better.

The "observe the symptoms of the addiction" step allows us to face any resistance to behaviors that support weight release. For many of us, this resistance is not only a deeply tangled neural net but also a genuine aversion to painful experiences. As previously shared, scientific studies have documented that adopting a mindfulness practice is tremendously helpful in developing new neural nets. However, despite the strong desire to release our extra weight, the resistance to practices such as meditation is rooted in our unwillingness to face our mental stories; in some cases, we are not even aware that there *is* a mental story. We encounter the same resistance when facing painful facts that we have repressed with lies. For example, we tell ourselves we don't have time to work out in order to mask the shame that we feel when we attempt to exercise.

Over the years, diets have enticed us by telling us that we don't have to change any of our mental stories, just eat something different. Wrong! Emotional eating is the trigger for most of our overindulging. Despite the stories diet programs have fed us for years (no pun intended), when our food triggers are emotional in nature, is not *what* we eat, but *why*.

We need to be willing to rewrite our stories according to our personal truth. Let's begin with that premise and consider the following:

I have at last arrived at a level of self-advocacy where I can face that persistent whisper that tries to convince me, "I don't have time to exercise." Those words are a lie. The truth is this: I HATED feeling like a whale while out jogging. I just knew everyone was looking at me in disgust. I was ashamed that I could not even run a city block. I felt painfully embarrassed that I could not keep up with the group during an exercise class. Furthermore, I convinced myself that others lost weight *without* any exercise.

Likewise the excuse that "I don't have time for things like meditation" is a lie. The truth is that every time that I attempted to meditate I experienced mixed emotions that I didn't understand. I wasn't able to admit to myself that I simply could not handle it. I got angry, anxious, or restless instead of getting peaceful. And I convinced myself that activities like meditation had nothing to do with losing weight.

Please document your reaction to the last two paragraphs. Are you:

- Ready to throw this book out the window?
- Completely in agreement with these statements?
- Experiencing a sudden anxiety attack or feeling restless or suddenly hungry?
- Curious as to how exactly something like meditation could help rewire your brain?
- All of the above?
- None of the above?

If you are experiencing anything that makes you so uncomfortable that you simply stop reading, let me restate that repression is the inability to face your stories. We fear anything that would disrupt our status quo.

If, after going through the whole list of what could possibly be fueling the emotional hunger, you can't identify with any of them, then you might have a deeply rooted belief that you are keeping yourself safe. It is then advisable to read books on repressed emotions, or attend Inner Child workshops, or talk with a therapist who has expertise in repressed emotions. All you need is the courage to start the exploration.

For me personally, 12-Step-type programs and Woody-Allen-like therapeutic relationships were never appealing. I felt that they substituted food addiction with therapy addiction. But I have finally acknowledged that what is important is for each one of us to find whatever allows us to arrive at self-acceptance and the ability to *embody* our feelings, not just *intellectualize* them. Once we are willing to look at our truth, the method is secondary. What is important is acknowledging our fears, as that obliterates the denial. The invitation in this addendum is for you to get in touch with what generates a sense of joy in your life. And yes, I fully understand that this is not an exercise that we are very adept at executing.

We need to accept that, for many of us, eating serves multiple functions beyond the act of providing nourishment to our body. If our denial is profound, then there is a wounded and terrified child inside us who is using overeating as a flawed attempt to soothe herself. The truth, however ugly, holds the freedom to transform overeating behavior.

We then arrive at the juncture where we are able to dismantle the biggest lie, the most damaging denial of all: the denial of our own inestimable power and value. The famous Marianne Williamson quote says, "Our deepest fear is not that we are inadequate, our deepest fear is that we are powerful beyond measure. It is our light, not our darkness that frightens us." Once we are awakened out of our addiction, we gradually, almost involuntarily, begin to act more like ourselves.

In some cases, overeating is an insidious form of self-hate. If you need to go to an Inner Child workshop, begin assertiveness training, or enroll in a class to improve communication skills, then make that investment in yourself! These outside programs might be necessary before you can "identify the real need" and name what is expressing itself as "emotional hunger." Remember, we are exhuming years of entrenched beliefs, and significant life changes might be necessary to ensure that the TCB protocol restores our Naturally Thin Woman behaviors.

Why Can't We Keep the Weight Off?

As we have repeatedly stated, once we become addicted to anything, emotional challenges will manifest as cravings for relief – in our case, for food. These challenges could be strong memories, attending a social function beyond our comfort zone, experiencing a highly enticing food commercial, even watching another person enjoying one of our forbidden foods.

The addict's thought process prioritizes short-term emotional relief over the long-term, rational benefits of sobriety. Until healthy neural nets have been re-established and emotional issues addressed, any trigger has the power to send us off on another binge.

The Compelling Nature of Emotional Hunger

Scientists describe addiction as a clash between brain systems, where balancing mechanisms go haywire, allowing pleasure/reward circuits to hijack the brain. Our food addiction has manifested because our brain is supposed to get a healthy dopamine boost every time we eat. We learn to not only associate eating with pleasure, but we crave that pleasure even when we are not physically hungry. Although there are healthier and less damaging ways to make ourselves feel better, a food-obsessed brain pushes us to eat in order to experience that pleasure again. It is a real and powerful force that conjures the mirage of pleasure and then propels us to consume much more food than we need to thrive. It is typically not accompanied by signs of physical hunger. It is an overwhelming, persistent, compelling obsession to experience *pleasure.*

So at the biological level the addiction is to the dopamine high. And learning how to keep that dopamine level healthy helps us to break the association of food as our primary source of pleasure.

As I previously shared, my history is one of being a neglected child. I used to believe that the way to nurture my inner little girl was to indulge her, to let her enjoy the sweets and other foods I craved, because she deserved that pleasure. It was transformational when I understood the huge difference between pleasure and shame.

Neglect is a painful experience for any adult but it is debilitating for a child. Overeating manifested in my life as *re-experiencing* the negative messages that I received as a child. "You are invisible. You are inconsequential. Your needs are unimportant. You have no worth. You have no value." When we believe that we don't belong, we feel compelled to achieve, to do anything within our talents in order to stand out and be recognized. We push ourselves to excel, since our intellect, our creativity, our fill-in-the-blank are things we quickly learn will garner our parents' approval. We become supremely good, peacemakers, or we're super-helpful, as that is one vehicle sure to make others need us.

I cried when I saw that my overeating was perpetuating the messages that I experienced as a child. It was healing, and a feeling of warmth bathed my soul. Only then was I able to understand the overeating behavior for what it was: an insidious form of self-rejection. It is critical to love ourselves, it is imperative to learn self-advocacy not as a to-do list, not as a facade, not as a meaningless battle cry, but as the ability to embrace the love that has eluded us for so long.

Love is fueled by emotions, but love is an *action*, and the most loving activity we can do for ourselves is to nurture ourselves with foods that contribute to our well-being in amounts that don't keep us weighted down.

The Addiction is to the Cycle of Shame

If you don't experience tangible progress as you attempt to build your new neural nets, try the following exercise:

1 – Next time you go on a full-blown binge, journal about what you feel *after* the binge. Give voice to the feelings that you experience after overeating, in detail. This is where self-knowledge and courage really count. You must be willing to be completely naked and vulnerable on paper.

2 – Identify where you adopted the beliefs that you felt after the binge: where did you learn those messages?

3 – Most psychotherapists will tell you that the addiction is not to the food, it is not to the pleasure, the addiction is to the cycle of shame; shame is a rush all unto itself. Shame is believing that we are not good enough, that our feelings don't matter, that our very existence is insignificant. We feel that we are not *deserving* of anything, and in many cases that we can only *earn* love.

How do you feel every time you overeat? How do you feel when you hear that the "addiction is to the shame"? Does it ring true for you at any level? If it does not, would you be willing to explore that possibility with a supportive person? If you choose a friend, they must have the courage to be with your pain and not run away from it. You want someone who is empathetic, who will not judge, condemn, or increase your sense of shame. If you can't think of any friends who have this degree of empathy, then seek counseling from a professional with expertise in the cycle of shame.

I went through a major catharsis when I realized that overeating was reinforcing my childhood belief that I was not good enough. Overeating was not indulging the little girl whose needs were seldom met. I was feeding the underlying, silent, inherent message that I did not matter. Food was my vehicle to be noticed, to feel *substantial*. At that moment of truth when the choice was to overindulge or nurture, I kept choosing to overindulge, as I simply did not have the self-advocacy to stand up to the emotional undertow.

The current paradigm for addiction has documented that when a child is raised feeling neglected and subsequently feels inadequate about herself, overeating becomes the vehicle to block/blot/cover/distract from the pain of feeling ashamed, and that destructive habit evolves into an addiction. Remove the deep-rooted shame, and we find the purpose, the strength, and the ability to stop our addictive, destructive overeating.

This one single exercise could be the Holy Grail in eradicating your overeating behavior. If your addiction is to the shame you feel after the binge experience – as it is for most addicts – then it is paramount to be willing to give up that shame.

Dr. Brené Brown, one of the leading researchers on the damage of shame, asserts that shame needs three things to continue to be a dominant force in our lives: secrecy, silence, and judgment. The unwillingness to effectively process our shame will keep the cycle growing and will manifest in our lives as the voracity of our appetite.

Ego Death

There is a quote from Dostoevsky that states, "The best way to keep a prisoner from escaping is to make sure he never knows he is in prison."

Most people assume that we feel *good* when we believe pleasant thoughts and *bad* when we believe unpleasant ones. This is partly true, but only when the pleasant thoughts are not deceptive. Mental stories are typically forged as protective armor against anything that is not congruent with our desires. Intractable emotional pain is always evidence that we believe something that is, at its core, false. Our willingness to dig into our traumatic history and to accept any present disappointments is the beginning of the healing journey.

I do not want to trivialize the ego death that must occur in order for us to accept our humanity and our flaws, completely and compassionately. It is challenging to exit a marriage that doesn't promote our well-being, especially if there are children involved. We fear that we may not be able to support ourselves or that we may have to give up our social status. The same is true if our current mental story keeps us in a job that is killing us, or convinces us to maintain relationships that are no longer nurturing, just because we believe that it is our obligation to be a good mother, daughter, friend, etc. We tend to embellish our mental stories when the truth threatens our status quo. On the other end of the spectrum, as Solzhenitsyn once said, "There are times when silence is a lie."

Thousands upon thousands of people have journeyed into the dark and uncomfortable cave to face their repressed emotions. With courage, love, and self-acceptance we can arrive at deeper levels of awareness where we can make peace with the imperfection of our humanity. Once we are congruent with our truth, the anxiety that drives us to overeat is gone and we can then clearly state:

- This is what I need.
- This is what makes me angry.
- This is how I'm feeling right now.
- This is how I want to be loved.

And it is not just insecure or timid people who use food as a shield; it is also the highly functional, super-achiever who shields her vulnerability at the cost of genuine love and honest feelings. This process is always challenging, always painful. The payoff, however, is that the energy we used to expend emotionally eating transforms into creativity, fascinating ideas, compassionate actions, and fantastic adventures. We must exit our mental stories and embody the emotions that we have learned to suppress with food.

The TCB protocol gives us the tools to face and deal with suppressed emotions without being shattered in the process. Start with:

- I want to eat, but I know that I'm not physically hungry.
- I recognize that I'm wired to crave food when there is an emotion that is begging for attention/resolution/release.
- I am willing to consider that I don't yet have the confidence to face whatever I have been repressing.
- I am ready to release the stories; I am ready to face whatever keeps me overeating.
- If during this process I become anxious, I recognize that I must seek support (perhaps even professionally) to help me identify what I'm repressing.

Personality Types

Warning: It is not our intention to oversimplify the complexity of different personality types. Entire books have been dedicated to each one of these. Instead, our hope is that readers who are ready to understand how their childhood experiences influenced their overeating behavior might find these summaries helpful. If you find yourself becoming anxious or getting defensive just reading these descriptions, consider that your reaction might be a form of self-protection. If you have the courage to explore some of these possibilities, please seek the help of wise friends or a professional counselor.

Let's review the history of how personality types develop and how they shape our coping strategies.

The Perfectionist/Super-Achiever Type – Many perfectionists adopt a strategy for creating order in the midst of chaotic family dynamics. They learn early in life that they can earn acceptance and attention from emotionally distant or demanding parents by standing out as the irreproachable, perfect child. High achievements can quiet the constant voice of self-judgment, and being outstanding leads to admiration from others – but it is a pseudo-form of love that brings only temporary relief. In many cases, perfectionism takes its toll as we neglect our health, pushing through fatigue by suppressing our personal needs and often eating to keep ourselves going.

Perfectionists experience constant frustration and disappointment with themselves and with others for not living up to impossible standards; this frustration is then stuffed with food. Perfectionists don't like dwelling on feelings for too long as they distract from achieving their goals.

For the Super-Achiever, self-validation, self-acceptance, and self-love are all predicated on performance. This is often the result of either conditional or altogether absent validation from parental figures. Even with very loving and approving parents, it is easy for children to get the sense that they are loved for their achievements, for obeying the rules, and for having good manners, rather than just for being themselves. When they feel empty or mildly depressed, they fail to acknowledge these emotions and instead stuff them with food.

My own story is that I used to feel worthy only when there was an external measure of success.

The Pleaser Type – If there is one personality that is disproportionately represented in the overweight population, it is the pleaser. Most pleasers earn attention and acceptance through helping others or being too responsive to others. Take for example the employee who constantly works weekends and overtime to please the boss, even to the detriment of her own health and personal life. These acts of selflessness are an indirect attempt to feed her emotional needs. This personality originates in three childhood assumptions:

1. I must put others' needs ahead of my own.
2. I must *give* love and affection in order to get any back.
3. I must earn love as I am not simply worthy of it.

We believe that expressing our needs is selfish, that we may drive others away. We are resentful about being taken for granted, but have difficulty expressing it. We don't recognize the source of these emotions; we experience "hunger" at the mere possibility of rejection.

The Victim Type – A victim is someone who feels powerless and is therefore unable to take appropriate action to resolve situations that adversely affect their well-being. Being powerless is a learned behavior originating from repeated childhood experiences where core needs were not adequately met. Victims tend to brood over negative feelings for a long time. They feel alone and lonely, even when they are around other people. Envy and negative comparisons abound. They go through life with black clouds over their heads and blame the world at large for their problems. Playing the victim is a strategy to squeeze affection or attention from the people who listen to the ongoing melodrama. The interaction between victim and audience mimics a sense of connection, but gives no real nourishment. Victims resort to food when their strategies do not garnish the attention that they are seeking.

The Mr. Spock Type – Young children often develop a hyper-rational survival strategy when there is emotional turmoil or chaos at home. They escape into an orderly, rational mind, generating a sense of security or intellectual superiority. This strategy also affords them attention and praise, since they show up as the smartest person in the room. Those of us who have adopted this facade are usually irritated when others get emotional, and we stuff that frustration with food. We become anxious about shielding personal time, energy, and resources against intrusions. We often feel different, alone, and not understood, but instead of expressing these feelings, we stuff them.

The High-Anxiety Type – High anxiety often comes from early experiences where the source of safety and security (the parental figure) was unpredictable, possibly due to addictions or personality disorders of their own. It can often result from painful events that "proved" life was threatening or unreliable. We feel skeptical, even cynical and are often anxious and hypervigilant. Food generates a sense of security and predictability that the rest of life does not offer.

The Restless Type – Restlessness is a strategy that urges us to find new sources of excitement, pleasure, and self-nurturing. This can be associated with early life experiences of inadequate parental nurturing. Indulgence in this strategy provides not only a substitute for nurturing, but also an escape from having to deal with anxiety and pain. The key characteristic is impatience with what is happening now and constantly wondering what is next. The restless personality fears missing out on any exciting experiences; they always want more and more. They worry that focusing on any unpleasant feeling will become overwhelming; one way to shift focus is to overeat.

The Controller Type – Underneath the bravado of the controller there is often a disturbing fear of being controlled by others or by life's events. The controller strategy is sometimes caused by early life experiences where the child is forced to grow up fast, be on her own, and take charge in order to survive physically and/or emotionally. It is also associated with being hurt, rejected, or betrayed and deciding never to be vulnerable again. Controllers experience high anxiety when things are not going their way. They experience anger and attempt to intimidate others who don't follow their commands. They are impatient with others' feelings and have low tolerance for different styles. They rarely admit feeling hurt or rejected, as that would mean that they had lost control. Food allows them to suppress these feelings.

The Avoider Type – The avoider can rise from either a happy or difficult childhood. With a happy childhood, one might not have had to develop the resiliency to deal with difficult emotions. In a childhood of high conflict and tension, the avoider develops from a need to restore peace and to mitigate negativity or tension. They value being even-keeled but then get anxious about what has been avoided. They also resent anyone who disturbs their peace and suppress their anger with food.

Belief Systems

The last day of an assignment where I had been consistently working 80-hour weeks, I reviewed my behaviors. No one had a gun to my head; it was a pattern I had repeated many, many times in my career, where I gave up my life for the success of the project. As with other projects, the price that I paid was my well-being, specifically the way that I dealt with my self-imposed deadlines and eating through the stress. When I fearlessly asked myself, "Why do I continue to engage in behaviors that don't serve me?" I discovered that it boiled down to what I believed:

1. I needed to be Superwoman to get these prestigious consulting assignments.
2. I needed to sacrifice, indeed suppress, my needs so that I could accomplish what I told myself must be achieved.

Behaviors are driven by thoughts that stem from beliefs. I'll give you a couple examples of my old beliefs, contrasted with what I now know is healthy:

Limiting Belief	Alternative Life-Enhancing Beliefs
I should be at the office as soon as I get up!	• Exercising first thing in the morning revs up my body, increases my vitality, relieves stress, improves focus, and *increases* productivity. • I'm evaluated by results, not by how many hours my butt is on the chair.

Limiting Belief	Alternative Life-Enhancing Beliefs
I need to constantly show how intelligent I am.	• Intelligence is leveraging the staff that I have. • Intelligence is taking care of myself. • Intelligence is empowering my staff to do their jobs.
Taking mini-vacations is too expensive.	• Removing myself from my day-to-day environment awakens all of my senses. It helps me feel renewed and fully alive. • What I do for a living is not measured in hours but in effectiveness. These investments in influence my overall efficiency, which benefits the project.

If we can't name what is masking itself as hunger, we might need to drill a little deeper and address the limiting beliefs that must be replaced by nurturing beliefs.

This page has been left blank intentionally.

Appendix B – Special Cases

Palate Reset

For women whose eating history involves mostly processed foods, there might be a need for a palate reset. Think about it: if you've mainly been eating foods that are substantially flavor-enhanced, the chemical additives have been directly stimulating your brain's pleasure center. Your palate will be challenged to detect when you are satisfied if it is competing with flavor enhancers that are programing your brain to eat more. Ditto if you are eating foods with elevated sugar content, as sugar is highly addictive.

To reset your palate, it will be necessary to eat foods that are not flavored-enhanced or processed for a minimum of four days. This will translate to eating only fruits, vegetables, grains, meats and non-processed cold cuts – in short, a diet with zero additives, as natural as possible.

After four days of eating in this manner, your ability to detect foods with high amounts of sugar, salt and other flavor-enhancers will be restored. This allows your palate to discern when you experience satiation.

Insulin-Resistant Women

Within three weeks of following the TCB program, most women report tremendous and perceptible progress, with one exception: women who are insulin-resistant. Insulin is the primary hormone that enables the body to absorb glucose, the key nutrient for many of our cells. Physiologically, these women's cells have become resistant to insulin, which inhibits their ability to absorb glucose nourishment and compromises the entire fueling mechanism.

Paradoxically, there is too much glucose in the blood, but their cells' ability to use that glucose has been compromised because the cells have ceased to obey insulin's instructions, and they stop absorbing a healthy amount of glucose. Insulin resistance can result from a genetic predisposition, but as the United States continues to experience epidemic level of diabetes, our food supply is suspected to be the primary cause of insulin resistance. Overconsumption of foods high in sugar and carbohydrates leads the body to produce more glucose than it can absorb. Even though there is a surplus of glucose in our bloodstream, the body starts craving more sugar and more carbs, which perpetuates a vicious cycle.

Characteristics and symptoms of women who are insulin-resistant include:

Adult acne	Heart palpitations
Anxiety	Hot flashes and night sweats
Bone loss	Insomnia or restless sleep
Breast pain	Irregular periods
Cravings	Irritability and mood swings
Digestive issues	Low libido
Dry skin	PMS
Fatigue	Stiffness or joint pain

Feeling depressed or overwhelmed	Unwanted hair growth
Fuzzy thinking	Urinary dysfunction
Hair loss	Vaginal dryness
Headaches	Weight gain

Women who are insulin-resistant are typically apple shaped (they hold most of their body fat around their stomach) and have at least eight symptoms from the previous list. Women who are insulin-resistant have extreme difficulty losing weight because part of insulin's function is to release fat to be used as fuel, but the body has stopped obeying insulin's instructions.

The good news is that insulin resistance is ***reversible***! Once you get your body to restore its insulin sensitivity, you will not only lose weight, but the many medical issues caused by insulin resistance (many of which require expensive drugs to manage) will be eradicated. The keys to the reversal are:

1. Managing your sugar and carb consumption
2. Withstanding the withdrawal symptoms
3. Managing stress
4. Weight training

Managing Sugar and Carb Consumption

When an insulin-resistant woman starts managing her blood-sugar level (first by eating five small meals a day that are rich in protein and good fats) and avoids all foods that have a high glycemic index, her body begins restoring insulin sensitivity. The recommended frequency with which you should fuel your body, how many grams of carbs and sugar your body can ingest at the same time, varies. Some health professionals suggest a maximum of 5 grams of sugar and up to 30 grams of carbs every 3 to 4 hours. It's not how many grams of sugar or carbs for the *entire day* but how many *at the same time*. A nice side effect of removing toxic quantities of sugar and carbs that your body can't handle is that insulin-resistant women begin to lose weight as the body re-establishes its ability to burn stored fat.

Eating every 3 or 4 hours can be challenging for a woman working outside the home, but it will help you avoid what now feels like an overwhelming drive to consume carbs and/or candy! Remember that a glass of low-sugar protein shake IS a meal! When you don't have time to prepare breakfast, drink a protein shake, but you must begin managing your blood-sugar level the moment you roll out of bed. Taking small sips of a protein shake during weight training is helpful, as it replenishes your protein level during/after muscle exhaustion.

Obviously the important part of restoring insulin sensitivity means eating foods low on the glycemic index: chicken, turkey, fish, eggs and managed amounts of red meat. This will probably mean clearing your pantry and refrigerator of everything that has added sugar. You will be shocked to discover how much sugar is added to 99% of all processed foods. The most effective plan is to get your carbs from fresh vegetables, and unfortunately, until you restore healthy insulin sensitivity in your body, most health professionals would recommend forgoing all fruits (a very small quantity of berries would fall within the guidelines, but it is a miniscule amount).

Withdrawal Symptoms

Women who are insulin-resistant crave sugar and carbs. Despite having too much glucose in the bloodstream, the body is starved for nutrients and wants sugar and carbs to satisfy the craving, but when that craving is satisfied it leads to a glucose spike.

Once you learn to become aware of this vicious cycle, you may feel as if you're surrounded by snipers; you have to be vigilant, because when your cells experience hunger, it will feel like an excruciating need for sugar or carbs – a bona fide episode of withdrawal symptoms, not unlike what drug addicts experience.

There are supplements that some individuals have reported helpful with these types of withdrawal symptoms: tyrosine, chromium, and glutamate are examples. There are also natural supplements that may help the body restore its insulin sensitivity: bitter melon, cinnamon bark, and *Gymnema Sylvestre* are examples of these. Some individuals find these supplements tremendously helpful in managing the withdrawal symptoms that you might experience as your body goes through its carb/sugar divorce and begins to restore its insulin sensitivity. And, as we outlined before, five small low-glycemic meals are the key to avoiding huge blood-sugar swings, and these supplements provide the safety net.

We recommend that you work with health professionals knowledgeable about managing withdrawal symptoms caused by sugar and carb cravings.

Managing Stress

The immune system plays a vital role in healing, and stress compromises your immune system's ability to heal. Cortisol is one of the hormones generated during elevated stress levels. High stress interferes with activities important for reversing insulin resistance, because cortisol causes more sugar to be generated by the liver, further decreasing the consumption of glucose by our cells. All of cortisol's actions block insulin function!

So know this, a body that is stressed out can't heal itself! As we have documented (and repeatedly nagged), meditation is not only fundamental to restoring our Naturally Thin Woman neural nets, it yields the highest return on investment for restoring insulin sensitivity because:

- it lowers your stress level, which directly helps restore insulin sensitivity
- it increases your dopamine level, which is helpful in withstanding your withdrawal symptoms
- it increases your sense of well-being, also helpful in managing your resources during this healing period.

If you eat flawlessly and exercise religiously but continue to live at a high stress level, it means that the nasty chemicals, especially cortisol, are still interfering with your body's ability to restore healthy insulin sensitivity. It is like building a house on a steep mountainside with no substructures to anchor it: all of that work slides down the hill the moment your stress level is elevated. Keep that perspective while you are restoring your insulin sensitivity. Nothing that causes stress is worth your health!!! Refer back to the section in Chapter 9 entitled "Stress-Proofing Your Brain" and invest in any activity that helps you manage your stress level.

Weight Training

The benefit of weight training in the prevention and treatment of insulin resistance is strongly supported by current research. Bigger muscles mean higher consumption of glucose, which your body needs. Additionally, building muscles releases hormones to help restore the health of insulin function. Marc Roig Pull, Ph.D., while at the University of British Columbia, ran a study that concluded: "Eccentric training performed at high intensities (with heavy weights, but not so heavy as to cause injury) [is] the most effective investment to build muscles."

To explain what eccentric training means, think about doing a bicep curl: when bend your arm to bring the weight up toward your shoulder (shortening the muscle), it's a concentric movement. When you *slowly* lower the weight back toward your thigh (lengthening the muscle), it's an eccentric movement. There are many YouTube videos you can watch to teach you how to perform these exercises.

The four major muscle groups are legs, chest, shoulders and back. Using heavy weights and focusing on eccentric exercises that target those four major muscle groups requires the lowest time investment and yields benefits to all of the muscles in the body. The reason is that these four muscle groups generate enough enzymes to help the rest of the muscles be restored to healthy levels. Weight training improves glucose levels because it reduces fat in the muscle, increasing muscle mass and the GLUT4 protein in muscle tissues, increasing insulin sensitivity.

Be aware of anything that might jeopardize your workout priorities! There will always be special meetings, work emergencies, demands that feel more important than your workout routine. Don't think of this as exercise, but rather an investment to optimize your health.

Restoring Insulin Sensitivity

As you restore healthy insulin sensitivities, many of the symptoms managed by prescribed medication will decrease. Work with your health professional to lower the dosage of these medications to correspond to the severity of your symptoms.

Finally, it is vital that you *measure progress and experience success* not only by what your scale says but also by how your clothes fit. As you weight train, you will be building your muscles, and the scale will not be the most effective tool to measure that progress, have someone take measurement of your body, so that you can track that progress.

If you think you might be insulin resistant, I would highly recommend working with your health professional. They can order a simple blood test to check your glucose level. In most major cities there are many laboratories that conduct these tests at reasonable prices. If your blood glucose level is high it should be baselined so that you can track its improvement, but you must review these results with a qualified health professional.

You have already baselined your weight, so yes, that can be tracked also. Beyond gauging these leading indicators, tracking the symptoms caused by insulin resistance (anxiety, hot flashes, depression, night sweats) will be highly beneficial. The combination of all of these factors will be irrefutable evidence that you are restoring a healthy level of insulin sensitivity.

These are all major life changes, but you know what's at stake here: your health, your vitality, your energy level, your joie de vivre, your passion for life, your productivity – in short, your ability to be the radiant, amazing woman whom you are meant to be! All of the medical symptoms that have plagued you while you were clueless that they were caused by insulin resistance will be finally and conclusively addressed, over, finito! It is time to reclaim a life of passion, creativity and loving relationships, and it starts by taking care of yourself.

Here is one of my all-time favorite quotes:

Don't ask what the world needs. Ask what makes you come alive, and go do it. Because what the world needs is people who have come alive.

Howard Thurman

Restore your brain and you contribute to the world!

This page has been left blank intentionally.

Index

Active Listening, 54
Active Meditation, 65, 70
Alexander, Bruce K., 24
American Medical Association, 40
American Psychiatric Association, 40
Anchors. *See* Neuro-Linguistic
    Programming
Antioxidants, 90
Aspartame, 37
Atkins, Robert C., 88
Attuned with Nature, 18, 24
Average Model, 39
Average Woman, 39
Ayurveda, 24

B6 Vitamin, 90
Ben-Shahar, Tal David, 105
Benson, Herbert, 63
Berridge, Kent, 49
Bitter Melon, 137
Blood Sugar, 18-19, 20, 47
Blues, The, 84
Blum, Kenneth, 27
Body Image, 38, 42
Boggiano, Mary, 30
Bolte-Taylor, Jill, 64
Boredom, 81, 84
Boston's Obesity Prevention Center, 38
Brain Differences, 29, 34
Brain Hunger, 16, 29, 45, 48, 52-53, 61,
    70, 95, 96
Brefczynski-Lewis, Julie, 63
Brown, Brené, 129

Calder, Andrew, 34
Carbohydrates, 38
CAT Scan, 16, 43
Caudate Nucleus, 49
Center for Disease Control, 57
Chamine, Shirzad, 66
Chew Slowly, 59
Childress, Anna Rose, 35
Chödrön, Pema, 106
Chromium, 137
Cinnamon bark, 137

Cognitive Behavioral Therapy, 43-44, 46,
    61, 63, 66, 104
CBT. *See* Cognitive Behavioral Therapy
Conscious Breathing, 60, 66, 85
Controller Personality, 132
Cornier, Marc-Andre, 34
Cortisone, 137
Cruise, Jorge, 88
Cycle of Shame, 86, 95-99, 103, 114-115,
    117, 128

Dahlström, Annica, 27
Dalai Lama, 64
DANA, 35
Depression, 82, 91
Deprivation, 23
Digestion, 24
Disappointment, 84-85
Dopamine, 27, 30-38, 42, 52, 59, 64, 68,
    106, 127, 137
Dopamine Receptors, 28, 30, 33
Dostoevsky, 129

Eat in Silence, 54, 58, 61
Eat Less, Move More, 10
Eccentric Weight Training, 138
EFS. *See* External Food Sensitivity
EFT. *See* Emotional Freedom Technique
Ego Depletion, 19, 53, 87, 106, 123
EMDR. *See* Eye Movement
    Desensitization and Reprocessing
Emotional Food Triggers, 47
Emotional Freedom Technique, 73, 75
Emotional Hunger, 56, 73-75, 77, 79-80,
    86, 114-115, 122-127
Emotional Imbalance, 25, 29, 34-35, 48,
    77, 80, 96-98, 113
Emotional Triggers, 34, 48, 55-56, 75, 95-
    99, 125, 127
Energy Meridians, 73
Enkephalins, 27, 38
Experiencing Success, 52
External Food Sensitivity, 47
Eye Movement Desensitization and
    Reprocessing, 72, 75

I said she seemed fine.

I'd meant to give her shin a fleeting inspection, but Val closed her eyes and let her head fall back and this gave me a chance to consider her neck. Or, more precisely, the soft hollow at the base of her neck where, in the final moment of release, the tendons seized up and the skin flushed with blood.

My fingers drifted up her shin and Val let her other leg sag open a bit.

"You should get going," she said.

"Right. Going."

"Because you said you had to go. And I want to respect that."

Val plucked at her dress. She did this sometimes, when she was nervous, the result being, in this case, that the hem rode up to the tops of her thighs. I could have accused her of subconscious sadism but she didn't believe in the subconscious. She would have said that she was hot, that she'd had too much wine, that I thought about these things too much.

"So anyway," she said. "Thanks."

She gave me a peck on the cheek. Then she leaned down to grab her camera and I could see her breasts struggling to free themselves, the prim pale bands that cut down from her shoulders and gracefully broadened above the nipple and the round outward swell, which made me want to suckle her, there in the fizzy yellow light of the front seat, in the motionless August night.

I reached for her thigh, the smooth expanse of the inner half, and she let out a shivery moan and we were going down once more, once more at least, in a tangle of black underwear and salty skin and dumb teenage lunging—the colliding teeth, the muscle spasms—and we didn't stop, couldn't stop, until I was all the way up inside and her ass was pounding the horn in a vibrant staccato. She looked how she always looked naked: she looked sautéed.

The problem, obviously, is that we were broken up. Not freshly, but a month or so in, during that phase when you're still trying to be pals— hey pal!—while also searching desperately for an excuse to leap into the sack. This wasn't the first time we'd backslid. It was more like the

third or, okay, the fourth. Fifth, I guess, if you count the day w[e] up, which, after all the tears and vows of sorrow, required that [we] standing up in the foyer of her apartment house.

Val and I had broken up mutually, and for all the right rea[sons. I] know how lame this sounds, but it's true. We weren't afraid of co[mmit]ment. We certainly didn't lack chemistry. But our personalities [didn't] square. She was one of those people lousy with sufficiency, the s[trong] silent type. I was more like the insecure loud type.

I made fusses in public, stiffed rude waiters, nearly wept a[t the] late-season ineptitude of the Red Sox. Val loved that I wasn't a[fraid] to show my feelings. And I marveled at her poise, the way she c[ould] soothe the people around her *without even speaking*. Even the way [she] shopped astounded me, the quiet dignity of her selections, bonel[ess] chicken thighs (from which she assiduously trimmed the fat), wh[ole] wheat tortillas, avocados only if ripe.

Eventually, though, my rants stopped seeming so funny. And h[er] silences began to grind me down. On long drives, I'd turn off the radi[o] and wait for her to say something, anything, a perfectly idiotic ploy fo[r] which I was invariably rewarded with the question: "Are you mad a[t] me?" But nobody was mad at anybody. That was the whole problem. We were just too stubbornly ourselves.

It would have been easier, I guess, if we'd had some big blowout. Or one of us had been unfaithful. But no, we were incompatible, a couple of crazy young incompatible horndogs panting through the endless sultry afternoons.

A week or so after the wedding, we met up at a free concert on the Common, the Boston Symphony doing Beethoven's Ninth—not exactly Barry White, but you take what you can get. The conductor was one of these old Japanese hipster dudes with a hairstyle like he'd just stuck his thumb in a socket.

Val was wearing cutoffs and a halter top. Was it inappropriate for me to slip my hand down the front of this garment during the rousing third movement (*adagio molto e cantabile*)? Or to blow warm air onto the nape of her neck as the woodwinds huffed out their mournful glissandos? Given that we were surrounded by ten thousand classical music nuts, many of

"Are you alright, sweetie?"

"I'm fine," she said softly. "Please take your hand out of my pants now, Mark."

I was on my way home from Wednesday night poker, where I'd lost forty bucks and drunk half that back. I could have taken a quicker route home. Sure. But the booze had done a number on my capacity for shame.

I sat in my car, staring up at Val's bedroom window, remembering how, on previous poker nights, she had met me at her door in silk pajamas. "Did you win us some money, honey?" she had asked me. "Are you going to buy us some jewels?"

We hadn't spoken since the concert, nearly a month ago, and I was certain she'd moved on by now, found a new guy to do the dirty work, a guy with a better job than me, a better wardrobe, and a bigger cock—sure, that was pretty much a no-brainer.

She sounded drowsy and annoyed on the intercom.

"Who *is* it?"

"Me."

There was a pause, an exhilarating juncture of doubt, and I felt sure she wasn't alone, that she was up there with Mr. Big New Cock, settling onto his lap with one of her impervious shudders.

Then I heard the metallic drone of the buzzer and leapt for the door and staggered upstairs. She was wearing an old T-shirt and a smug look, as if she'd known this was coming all along.

"Just in the neighborhood?" she said.

"Poker."

She sniffed at me. "Poker and liquor. How novel. You really know how to make a girl feel special."

"It's not like that," I said.

"Tell me how it's like."

We were standing in her front room. The door to her place was open. The light from the hallway made her split ends glow like filaments.

"I was just thinking about you, that's all. Wondering how you were doing."

"How sweet."

"Am I doing something stupid here? You can tell me if I'm doing something stupid, Val."

"You're doing something stupid."

I nodded.

She yawned and reached to cover her mouth and her shirt rose to reveal her panties, the darkened triangle that stood out against the white cotton. "You really are a piece of work," she said.

"Okay," I said. "Total jerk move. I plead guilty to whatever, to nostalgic lechery in the first degree. You can release me on my own recognizance."

"I wish it were that simple," Val said. Her grin thickened into something sort of menacing. "No, I think we'll need to take care of your punishment right now."

I heard footsteps in the other room and for a second I waited for her new guy to emerge, naked and spoiling for a fight. But the noise was just a poltergeist conjured up by my puny conscience.

Val settled back against the wall and slipped her right hand under the waistband of her panties. Oh, that soft wet clicking! Those nimble fingers! And how she spoke to me, in urgent puffs, as I stood there stiffening up: "You want to see how I'm doing, huh? You want to make sure I'm not too lonely? That my little *concha* isn't too lonely? Mmmmm. Oh no, don't touch, baby. That's not for you to touch. That's not yours anymore, remember? Mmmm. All this over here, all this wet stuff, that's not for you anymore."

Concha? I'd never heard her speak this way. Had she been fucking a Latin guy? Was that what this was about? Some Cuban-variety bohunk who had uncaged the vixen within her using his all-powerful *pingote?*

Val's breathing had grown raspy and her thighs were pulsing and her hand, swirling there beneath her panties, looked like a lurid little sock puppet.

What was I supposed to do? Just stand there in my drunken lust and *watch?* I loosened my belt and let my pants settle around my ankles. Val pulled her hand out of her panties and stepped toward me and ran her finger under my nose. Then she took hold of my shirt collar and I felt my feet go out from under me and my hip banged against the wood floor. I watched from below as Val swung the door to her place shut.

She lowered herself onto my chest. Her knees came to rest on my